WHAT TO DO IF YOU GET COLON CANCER

Also by Marian Betancourt:

What to Do if You Get Breast Cancer
Chronic Illness and the Family: A Guide for Living Every Day

Also by Paul Miskovitz:

The Evaluation and Treatment of the Patient with Diarrhea

WHAT TO DO
IF YOU GET
COLON CANCER

A Specialist Helps You
Take Charge and
Make Informed Choices

Paul Miskovitz, M.D., and Marian Betancourt

John Wiley & Sons, Inc.

New York · Chichester · Weinheim · Toronto · Singapore· Brisbane

Library of Congress Cataloging-in-Publication Data

Miskovitz, Paul F.
  What to do if you get colon cancer : a specialist helps you take charge and make informed choices / Paul Miskovitz, Marian Betancourt.
    p.   cm.
  Includes bibliographical references and index.
  ISBN 0-471-15984-0 (pbk. : alk. paper)
  1. Colon (Anatomy)--Cancer--Popular works.   I. Betancourt, Marian.
II. Title.
RC280.C6M57   1997
616.99'4347--dc21   97-10074

Printed in the United States of America

10 9 8 7 6 5 4 3 2

For our families

CONTENTS

INTRODUCTION

The principles of colon cancer treatment have not changed since the nineteenth century, but the techniques of treatment have advanced light years. Some of the most dramatic advances came in the 1970s with the development of fiberoptic endoscopic instruments that allowed doctors to see inside the digestive system. Before that, colon cancer discovery at an early stage was more difficult. Another breakthrough came in 1989 when a particular combination of chemotherapy drugs dramatically improved survival rates of colon cancer patients with a particular stage of the disease.

When former President Ronald Reagan reported the removal of polyps from his colon in the 1980s, the public became aware for the first time of the importance of early detection. If polyps were found and removed early, colon cancer could be prevented. In some communities, people began lining up at their gastroenterologists' doors, sometimes having to wait several weeks for a colonoscopy, a relatively straightforward endoscopic procedure for viewing inside the colon.

Colon cancer evolves from a precancerous benign lesion or polyp that is allowed to remain in the large intestine and grow. The goal of colon cancer prevention is to interrupt that process and to find and remove the polyp or tumor before it becomes cancerous. Or, if it is in the early stage of becoming cancerous, the patient can be cured before the cancer has a chance to spread. The majority of colon cancers detected by screening programs are cured. Yet only half of all colon cancer cases are diagnosed at the curable stage. If we can only convince more people to get regular screenings, such as an annual digital exam, fecal occult blood test, complete blood count, periodic sigmoidoscopy, and, in selected patients, colonoscopy, we can knock colon cancer off the list of killers.

It has been estimated that half the population over age 50 have colon polyps, and 95 percent of colon and rectal cancers originate with such polyps. We know this from autopsy studies, which also show that the number of polyps found varies widely among regions of the world. Several European countries have higher rates than the United States, but in most developing nations, the rate is considerably lower. In the United States, the incidence of colon cancer is greater in the north and in the east and lower in the south and in the west.

Colon cancer and rectal cancer are major health problems in the United States with almost 200,000 new cases diagnosed each year. They kill nearly 60,000 Americans every year. In adult men, these cancers are second in prevalence only to lung cancer. In adult women, they are the third most prevalent cancers after breast cancer and lung cancer. The good news is that, while the number of cases is increasing, the mortality rate is decreasing, indicating that early detection is becoming more widespread.

According to 1996 statistics from the American Cancer Society, deaths from colon and rectal cancer combined declined 9 percent in men and 31 percent in women from 1962 to 1992. However, in separating colon cancer and rectal cancer, there was a 10 percent increase in deaths from colon cancer for men, but the deaths decreased 24 percent in women. Both men and women saw a decrease by more than half during that period in deaths from rectal cancer.

Treatment for colon cancer does not offer the patient as many options as does prostate cancer or breast cancer. A woman with breast cancer can make informed choices on whether to have a mastectomy or lumpectomy. A man with prostate cancer can choose the wait-and-see approach or can have his prostate removed. With colon cancer, the only option is to remove the cancer, whether it is confined to a polyp or has spread into the colon wall.

Nevertheless, colon cancer patients do have options. One option is to choose only those doctors and medical centers where they feel confident of getting the best treatment and follow-up care. Another option is to hear the truth about diagnosis and treatment and how treatment will affect a patient's lifestyle and future—and his or her family. In other words, patients have the option to become *informed* and to take charge of their health care.

If you are a colon cancer patient, you will learn, in this book, what your treatment is and is not. We will walk you through the process so you will have a guide, a way to understand what your physicians are advising, how to know what questions to ask, and what you should expect from your treatment and the healthcare professionals.

We have made special effort to alert you to particular points in the treatment process that might be compromised if you are insured by a healthcare program that might limit your treatment choices. We hope that *What to Do if You Get Colon Cancer* will help you know what to ask your doctors and where to get information and treatment with which you feel confident.

It is our hope that you will get the best treatment possible and that you will spread the message about early detection. If everybody will get early screenings for colon cancer, we can forever eliminate its threat to life.

ACKNOWLEDGMENTS

Our sincere thanks to physicians and other healthcare professionals who shared their expertise on colon cancer treatment and patient care, including Joseph Ruggiero, M.D.; Roger Yurt, M.D.; J. Francois Eid, M.D.; Marcus Loo, M.D.; Peter Farano, M.D.; Georgeanne Yurtin, R.N., M.S. Special thanks to literary agent Vicky Bijur.

PART I

DISCOVERY

1

WHAT YOU NEED TO KNOW ABOUT COLON CANCER

When our hearts are not working, we feel a pain in the chest or shortness of breath. We *know* when something is wrong. But when something is wrong with the colon, we can be unaware of it for years. And even when we have symptoms, it is easy for a patient—or even a less than diligent healthcare provider—to blame it on other conditions, such as diverticulosis, colitis, hemorrhoids, or irritable bowel syndrome.

Because vague abdominal discomfort is so commonplace, the symptoms of colon cancer can often be confused with those of benign conditions, and patients sometimes fail to pursue thorough diagnostic screenings. It is far easier to diagnose a patient who has had a regular bowel movement at the same time every morning for 40 years and now, for some reason, is having a different experience. Something tangible must have caused that change. But the patient who has always had bowel problems is going to be more difficult to diagnose. Even those previously treated for colonic ailments identified as benign are not protected from the development of colon cancer.

Although the title of this book is *What to Do if You Get Colon Cancer*, we are really talking about rectal cancer, colorectal cancer, and colon cancer—they are all the same disease. When we use the words *colon cancer,* we mean any cancer in the colon—from the cecum, at the beginning of the colon, to the rectum, the lowermost

3

portion of the colon. (Because of the location of the rectum, treatment is sometimes different.)

In order to understand how you got colon cancer and how treatment will affect you, it is important to understand the role of the colon in the mechanics of the digestive system. If you are going to need surgery for colon cancer, your entire digestive system will be shut down for several days, and understanding how that system works will better prepare you to cope with all the procedures involved in your treatment and follow-up care.

A GUIDE THROUGH THE DIGESTIVE SYSTEM

The digestive system sends us messages all the time. Our stomachs growl when we are hungry. We feel a burning sensation in our esophagus or stomach when we eat something irritating. We feel a knot in our stomach when we are upset. We might have a gut reaction to some encounters in our lives. We get a very particular urge when we have to go to the bathroom. All of these signals come from a complex system of dynamics that involves our entire physiology—blood, nerves, hormones, muscles—and its interaction with the brain.

A series of involuntary wavelike muscle contractions propels your food in one direction along the alimentary tract—from the mouth to the anus. This action is called *peristalsis*. When your stomach gurgles, it is the sound of these peristaltic contractions propelling food along, an action that you cannot feel. In the stomach, peristalsis produces a churning action that aids digestion. Circular muscles called *sphincters* are located at the entrance to the esophagus and at the exits from the esophagus, the stomach, the lower small intestine, and the rectum, or anal opening. These muscles close tightly to prevent the process from going in reverse and causing one to vomit.

On its trip through the alimentary tract, food is broken down into small molecules. Starches become simple sugars. Fats change to fatty acids and glycerine. Proteins become amino acids. The salivary glands in the mouth produce lubrication and begin this conversion. The stomach stores and digests about one quart of food, which muscles churn and mix with gastric juice, which includes hydrochloric acid and pepsin.

Within two to five hours, the digested food passes from the stomach to the *duodenum,* the first section of the small intestine. The *small intestine* is a 20-plus-foot-long, narrow, muscular tube—like a coiled soft-rubber hose—that is made up of layers called the *mucosa,* the *submucosa,* and the *serosa.* The main function of the small intestine is to secrete digestive juices into the digestive tract. Also, enzymes from the pancreas, alkaline juices, and bile emulsifiers made by the liver and stored in the gall bladder enter the system at the duodenum level. Bile acids help dissolve (solubilize) dietary fats the way detergent dissolves grease in dishwater.

Most absorption, as well as digestion, occurs in the small intestine. Nutrients are absorbed into lymph fluids or blood vessels in the intestine wall (across the mucosa). Whatever cannot be digested in the small intestine, such as plant fiber, empties into the cecum at the lower right side of the abdomen. The *cecum* is the beginning of the *large intestine*—or colon. The colon is shorter than the small intestine—only about 5 feet long—but it is much wider (the girth is responsible for the label *large* intestine). The colon partially encircles the small intestine.

The main function of the large intestine is to absorb salt and water from all the remaining digested food that has been passed from the small intestine. In a healthy adult, more than a gallon of water, with more than an ounce of salt, is absorbed from the colon every four hours. Bacteria in the colon then convert fecal matter into its final form.

Digested matter travels upward from the cecum into the ascending colon, across the abdomen in the transverse colon, down the left side of the abdomen in the descending and sigmoid colon, and into the rectum, where the solid waste is stored until it is eliminated. In doing this job, the colon produce a variety of substances, including carbon dioxide, hydrogen, methane, and the billions of bacteria that live in the colon.

All of this coiled tubing is supported by the *mesentery,* a membranelike fold of tissue attached to the back of the abdominal wall. The mesentery contains blood vessels, nerves, and the lymph system that interacts with the intestines.

Digestion and the absorption of nutrients into the bloodstream are as effortless as breathing, and normally, produces no sensations like pain. Most discomfort in the gastrointestinal tract occurs in the two main storage areas: the stomach and the colon. When you feel discomfort above the waist, it is often in your esophagus or stomach, both close to the heart. Thus, indigestion is often called heartburn. Discomfort below the waist usually means a problem in the colon, such as constipation or diarrhea.

HOW POLYPS FORM
IN THE COLON

A polyp is a new growth of tissue that serves no purpose. This kind of growth can occur in the inner lining of the colon when the cells in the mucous membrane—epithelial cells—for some reason fail to adhere to their normal routine. This abnormal growth can be caused by genetic programming or by years of wear and tear on the colon. Polyps can grow inside the colon for years without being noticed. All polyps in the colon are either benign or malignant and should be removed. Benign polyps are always removed—to make sure they are benign—because it is believed that if they stay in the colon long enough, they might become cancerous.

Again, think of the colon and rectum as a long hollow tube or pipe, the inner lining of which is called the *mucosa*. Polyps and cancers arise from this mucosal lining. A polyp is a protrusion into the *gut lumen* (the passageway inside the colon) of a small amount of mucosal tissue. When discovered by barium enema X ray, colonoscopy, or sigmoidoscopy or during surgery, polyps are always measured by their greatest dimension in millimeters (25.4 millimeters = 1 inch).

Polyps are sometimes further described as sessile or pedunculated, depending upon their shape. *Sessile polyps* have a broad base and are often only slightly raised above the mucosa, whereas *pedunculated polyps* are attached to the mucosa by a narrow stalk.

Although polyps of the colon might contain cancer within them, the word *polyp* usually refers to a benign condition. (Polyps attach to the mucosa, but unlike cancers they do not "invade" through the mucosa.) When removed and examined after proper processing and staining under the light microscope by pathologists, polyps can be further classified by the appearance of their cells and their architecture as *adenomatous, hamartomatous, hyperplastic,* or *inflammatory.* These last three, while unusual, are not considered precancerous. Most authorities believe it is the adenomatous polyp that is precancerous through a mechanism known as the adenoma-carcinoma sequence. Adenomatous polyps can be further subclassified by their histologic appearance into *tubular, villous,* or *tubulovillous* types.

Over 95 percent of cancers of the colon are thought to originate in a polyp, and the risk of an adenomatous polyp of the colon or rectum containing cancer appears to be, in part, directly dependent upon its size. For polyps less than 1 centimeter (about one-third of an inch or the size of a small pearl), the risk of cancer appears to be between 0 and 2 percent. For those polyps that measure 1 to 2 centimeters (up to three-quarters of an inch or the size of a large grape), the cancer risk appears to be between 10 and 20 percent. Polyps over 2 centimeters hold a cancer risk of 30 to 50 percent. Cancer is also more likely to develop in villous adenomas than in tubular adenomas or tubulovillous adenomas. However, some adenomas might never grow and become malignant.

Benign polyps might simultaneously coexist with cancer elsewhere in the colon and rectum. These are known as *synchronous lesions.* If a polyp is discovered during flexible fiberoptic sigmoidoscopy, which sees the lower third of the colon, it is good medical practice to then examine the entire colon with colonoscopy, a similar procedure that uses a longer instrument, to discover any simultaneously occurring polyps or cancers. In general, someone with a tendency to form colonic or rectal polyps is also at a higher risk of developing colon and rectal cancer.

Most patients who have polyps have no symptoms to warn of their presence. Thus, polyps are likely to remain undiscovered and undiagnosed until the colon and rectum are inspected by colonoscopy or barium enema X ray. In rare cases, polyps might cause occult, or hidden, amounts of blood to appear in the stool or might actually cause hemorrhage from the anus. Even more rarely, patients might complain of abdominal discomfort when a polyp stalk is subjected to peristaltic action (digested matter passing through) and "tugs" at the colon wall. If the polyp is very large, usually in the several-centimeter range, a blockage of the colon or rectum might occur and cause a person such distension or discomfort that it comes to the attention of a physician.

Three-quarters of adenomatous polyps and cancers are found in the left, or sigmoid, colon. Left-sided adenomas are more likely to be detected by fiberoptic endoscopy, and naturally are more likely to come to a physician's attention. However, the frequency of many smaller adenomas in the right colon, which can only be seen with colonoscopy, increases with age, especially after 60.

INSIDE THE COLON WALL

The lining of the colon undergoes constant regrowth of cells and renews itself completely every week. This process of cell growth— *proliferation* and *differentiation*—is highly regulated. Cells are produced, they mature, and they die at a regulated pace, so that the lining of the colon remains at the same thickness and maturity with a healthy mix of cell types.

However, when the cells disregard this process and begin to multiply and change character, the lining of the colon changes, and this can be observed endoscopically. Now the lining, or epithelium, has a characteristic look called *dysplasia.* This means the epithelial cells are not behaving normally. This can be an early sign of malignancy and always raises a red flag to the gastroenterologist and pathologist. Polyps with severe dysplasia can become malignant in less than four years.

Another change that can be observed is *hyperplasia,* the excessive growth of a single layer of cells, which becomes several cell layers thick. Although the cells are not malignant, they are atypical and could change. Because these conditions indicate unusual cell activity, they must be treated with the same thoughtfulness as true colon cancers. Premalignant conditions can remain localized (contained within an area) until they develop into either noninvasive cancer or invasive cancer. Then there is the potential for spread into surrounding tissue or even the rest of the body. Hyperplastic polyps are not premalignant but cannot be diagnosed as "hyperplastic" until they are removed and biopsied.

ADENOCARCINOMAS

Exactly how the polyp progresses to cancer still is not known, but most polyps seem to take from three to seven years to become malignant. The potential for the polyp to become cancer depends on its size and type, and degree of *atypia*. This is why regular screenings are so important. These polyps should be found and removed before they become cancerous. Some polyps are small with low-grade cell growth and pose no immediate danger. Others are fast growing and aggressive and can spread to other organs.

The chance of a polyp becoming cancer increases two and a half to four times if the polyp is larger than one centimeter—or one-third of an inch—in diameter. The chance increases five to seven times if multiple polyps are present. The natural history of a polyp larger than 1 centimeter left untreated shows that the progression to cancer increases 2.5 percent at 5 years, 8 percent at 10 years, and 24 percent at 20 years. This progression depends also upon the degree of dysplasia, or what the cells are doing. With severe dysplasia, the progression can be as little as 3.5 years, and with mild dysplasia, it might take more than 11 years.

Patients who have one adenoma are 30 to 50 percent more likely to have at least one more somewhere in the colon. Because multiple primary lesions (polyps, adenomas) occur so often, a total colonoscopy is an essential part of the workup if a lesion is found during a more limited exam. If there are multiple lesions in the colon, they are generally *synchronous lesions*—those that occur simultaneously—or *metachronous lesions*—those that occur at different times. These can be near one another or located in different parts of the colon.

People with familial polyposis syndromes, ulcerative colitis, or a previous history of colon cancer are more likely to have synchronous polyps. Patients with at least two synchronous adenomas are also more likely to have metachronous adenomas, that is, they are at increased risk to develop more polyps later. Part of the importance of finding and removing a polyp is that the physician has identified a patient who will need surveillance for early detection of additional polyps and possibly colon cancer.

9

In Situ or Invasive Cancer

Cancer is either in situ or invasive. *In situ* means "in place," contained within the polyp. The cancer has not broken through the colon wall into the surrounding muscle and fat. Thus, it is noninvasive.

Invasive, or infiltrating, cancer *can* break through or *already has* broken through the stalk of the polyp or through the colon wall into blood vessels, the lymph system, surrounding fatty tissue, or other organs.

If the cancer is invasive, lymph nodes around the colon must also be examined to find out if the cancer has begun to spread elsewhere. Lymph fluids flow through the body like the bloodstream, and the bean-shaped lymph nodes are like filters, catching what comes through the pipes. As part of the immune system, they filter out and get rid of foreign or abnormal cells. It is here that colon cancer cells are likely to travel on their way to other organs.

Metastatic Cancer

Metastatic means the cancer has spread through the lymphatic system or the bloodstream to adjacent and/or distant tissues. Sites of local metastasis of colon cancer are usually lymph nodes. The liver and lungs are the most common site of distant metastasis, followed by the adrenals, the ovaries in women, and then bone. Metastasis to the brain is rare.

Other Cancers That Rarely Occur in the Colon

Lymphomas can cause lymph nodes to enlarge and form a mass in the colon. Sometimes what appears to be an adenomatous polyp in the colon is not colon cancer at all, but cancer of the lymph system. The cancer can be *primary*—starting in the lymphatic tissue in the abdomen—or *systemic*—the colon mass is only one of the lymphoma tumors throughout the body. Colonic lymphomas account for less than 0.5 percent of all colonic malignancies and are treated differently than colon cancers.

Sarcomas are rare malignancies that might arise from the colon lining. Kaposi's sarcoma has become more common with the emergence of AIDS and appears as a complication of that disease, involving about 75 percent of AIDS patients. The stomach and duodenum are more common sites for these sarcomas, but about one-third of patients also get them in the colon.

There are also other rare tumors that appear in the colon or rectum, including colloid carcinoma, signet ring cell carcinoma, adenosquamous carcinoma, and oat cell carcinoma.

UNDERSTANDING THE RISK FACTORS FOR COLON CANCER

Most cancer of any kind can be defined as an acquired genetic disease produced by exposure to environmental carcinogens that cause damage that accrues over many years. Everyone is exposed to environmental carcinogens—cigarettes, gasoline, pesticides, radiation. Colon cancer is a multistage process, and the passage of time is needed for these chance events to accumulate and produce the genetic mutations that cause the cancer.

In the United States, where one in four deaths is from cancer, men have a one-in-two lifetime risk of developing cancer, and women have a one-in-three risk. *Lifetime risk* is the probability that anyone over the course of a lifetime will develop cancer or die from it. However, relative risk must also be considered. *Relative risk* is a measure of the relationship between risk factors and a particular cancer, and it increases with exposure to particular environmental elements, or with an inherited predisposition. Smokers, for example, have 10 times the relative risk of developing lung cancer than nonsmokers do. And a woman with a first-degree relative with breast cancer has twice the risk of developing that cancer.

Medical-history taking is extremely important. Most physicians like to make a clear distinction between patients at risk for colon cancer because of age and those patients with diseases that predispose to colorectal cancer.

Additional risk factors include a personal history of colonic or rectal polyps, a family history of such polyps, a personal or family history of colon or rectal cancer, and certain other bowel and nonbowel conditions. The lifetime risk of an adult developing colon or rectal cancer is about 5 percent. From this baseline, a number of risk factors can be identified.

Aging

The mere act of aging enhances the likelihood of getting colon cancer. By the age of 40, the number of people getting this cancer each year begins to accelerate, doubling every decade until about age 80. For the majority—about 70 percent—of patients diagnosed with colon cancer, the only risk factor they have is their age. Age is the major determinant in frequency of colon cancer, with peak prevalence in men and women after the age of 60.

The Family Gene Pool

When someone has lung cancer, the first thing a doctor will ask is whether the person smokes. If someone has leukemia, the doctor asks about exposure to radiation. With bladder cancer, the question is about exposure to industrial chemicals. But the first thing asked of a patient who has colon cancer is whether or not anyone in the family has had colon or rectal cancer.

In addition to the rare cases of hereditary colon cancer syndromes such as familial polyposis, there is more and more evidence that heredity plays a major role in the development of colon and rectal cancer. The probability of colon cancer developing in a person who has a first-degree relative with this cancer is about 15 percent, as compared to a 5 percent risk in the general adult population. Studies have shown that patients with colonic polyps are two to five times more likely to have a first-degree relative with colon polyps. And those first-degree relatives are two to five times more likely to have colon cancer than the general population.

The National Polyp Study, lead by scientists at Memorial Sloan-Kettering Cancer Center in New York, concluded in 1996 that siblings and parents of patients with adenomatous polyps are at increased risk for colon cancer, particularly when the adenoma was diagnosed before the age of 60, or in the case of siblings, when the parent has had colon cancer. Data from this study are expected to provide a basis for planning family-screening strategies. (Chapter 19 deals with protecting the family members of a colon cancer patient from developing colon cancer.)

Preexisting Bowel Conditions

It is well documented that colon and rectal cancer can occur as a complication of chronic ulcerative colitis and to a lesser extent Crohn's disease. This is particularly so if the disease began early in life and has been present for over 15 years.

- **Chronic ulcerative colitis (CUC)** is the inflammation of part or sometimes all of the colon. Ulcerative colitis most often occurs between the ages of 15 and 35 and begins in the rectum and progresses through the colon, which then becomes inflamed and ulcerated. This disease causes episodes of bloody diarrhea. It is often painful and can be accompanied by loss of appetite and weight. Severe ulcerative colitis could perforate the colon or could cause anemia and other complications. The cause of CUC is unknown, but it is a disease of Western countries—rare elsewhere. A milder and more common form of colonic ailment is irritable bowel syndrome (spastic colon), which is *not* considered a risk for colon cancer.

  Approximately 5 percent of CUC patients will get colorectal cancers, and the longer they have this disease, the greater the risk. CUC patients tend to be younger than the ordinary colon cancer patient at the time of diagnosis. For patients with CUC, it has been shown that the cumulative probability of developing colorectal carcinoma is 3 percent at 15 years, 5 percent at 20 years, and 9 percent at 25 years. Sixty percent of the people with CUC of the entire colon for more than 30 years will get colon or rectal cancer.

  Patients with CUC should have annual surveillance colonoscopy. In addition, they should have multiple biopsies of the colonic mucosa beginning 7 years after the onset of universal colitis and 15 years after the onset of left-sided colitis. The biopsy specimens should be examined under the microscope by pathologists for the presence of precancerous changes called dysplasia. Dysplasia is rated by a grading system as being either absent, low-grade, moderate-grade, or high-grade. When high-grade dysplasia is found, a total proctocolectomy—the removal of the entire colon and rectum—is usually called for.

- **Crohn's disease** is sometimes known as *enterocolitis,* and about 2 percent of patients with this disease eventually get colon cancer. For these patients, the findings are not as dramatic as those for CUC but are still higher than simple age-related risk. This group is usually older than the patients with CUC and is more likely to have multiple primary lesions. Crohn's disease also appears to be more common in men.

- **Diverticulitis** is *not* considered a risk factor for colon cancer, but it is mentioned because the symptoms are often very similar, and so is the treatment. When ballooned sacs are forced outward on the colon wall, this is called *diverticulosis.* When they become inflamed, these pouches can burst and spread bacteria into the abdominal cavity. In the worst case scenario, this can cause peritonitis and death. Treatment is similar to that for colon cancer, in that the diseased section of the colon often must be removed and resected after the administration of antibiotics.

Nonbowel Conditions

Genital and breast cancer in women have been proposed as risk factors for the development of colorectal cancer. Although there is no absolute proof of this connection yet, many physicians—especially oncologists—advise such patients to get regular screenings with sigmoidoscopy or colonoscopy.

Diet, Environment, and Race

Whether or not environment and diet are important risk factors for colon cancer remains to be proven, but they are taken into consideration because of the studies suggesting that geography and diet might factor into the *incidence* of colon cancer. For example, colon cancer risk is higher in African-Americans than it is in native black African populations, suggesting again the impact of environmental factors. But is it genetic or environmental? Or both? Colon cancer incidence is low in Japanese men, but when these men move to Hawaii, the incidence of colon cancer increases dramatically. Is it the dietary switch from fish and rice to bacon cheeseburgers?

There is still no positive proof that diet—such as high-fat, low-fiber—alone is responsible for colon cancer. This is still being investigated. It is known that a low-fat, high-fiber diet is generally more healthful and prevents digestive problems, as well. It appears that people who consume high amounts of fiber and who have large, bulky stools tend to have lower frequency of colon adenomas and cancers possibly because waste matter moves through the colon faster. But it still is not known which types of fiber are involved and how much needs to be consumed.

Lack of dietary calcium has also been studied as a risk factor on the theory that calcium and vitamin D neutralize fatty acids created by the high-fat diet—much the way detergent cuts the grease in the dishwater—and slows epithelial cell growth. Aspirin and related compounds are also under study, but the dynamics of the digestive system are too complicated for easy answers. For instance, the bacteria flora in the colon might oxidize bile acids that may have tumor promoting activity. It will be years before studies produce hard facts on this area. (For more information about diet and colon cancer, see Chapter 15.)

IDENTIFYING THE SYMPTOMS

Because there are so many symptoms of colon diseases that overlap with colon cancer, it is easy to confuse the issue or to try to second guess unless careful and methodical testing is done. More than a third of colon cancer patients studied had no symptoms. Symptoms usually do not occur until polyps become larger than one centimeter—about the size of your smallest fingernail—or until they crowd each other, as in the multiple polyps associated with familial polyposis syndromes. Symptoms like constipation, diarrhea, flatulence, and painful bowel movements can also be symptoms of ulcerative colitis, irritable bowel syndrome, or diverticulosis.

A patient who has an annual physical and discovers anemia, for example, must identify the cause. It could range from blood loss from taking too many aspirins to menstruation. No problem is obvious. A doctor is faced with a host of questions here and must rule out all other possibilities before making a diagnosis. First, the patient is questioned about possible reasons for loss of blood: Were there any changes in diet? In bowel habits? Could bleeding be caused by hemorrhoids, ulcerative colitis, or diverticulitis? The doctor must tease out suspicions from new onset anemia and make the patient understand why further—and more invasive—tests are necessary.

Laura, a woman in her 60s, went to Egypt with three friends and took a cruise through the Nile region. All four women suffered from diarrhea, which they attributed to the food and water in their new environment. But while the other three women got better when they returned home, Laura did not. After listening to her account of what was wrong, the doctor had to ignore the travel story and look beyond that. Then through careful questioning, examination, and screening, it was found that Laura had colon cancer. It was only a coincidence that it developed at the time of the cruise.

Audrey Hepburn, the actress and humanitarian, who died of colon cancer, was working in Africa, where the incidence of intestinal distress is not unusual because of the conditions of the water and the diet. One would not give a second thought to such symptoms. This is why it is so important to do so much testing before making a diagnosis.

June, a 75-year-old woman, experienced vague abdominal discomfort and some constipation, but because she had been overindulging in food and wine during the holidays, she assumed her gastric discomfort was related to that. She took antacids, hoping to feel better. When she finally had a checkup, a malignant tumor was discovered high up in her colon, in the cecum.

When colon cancer is located in the right side of the colon, the cecum, the most common symptomatic complaints are abdominal pain that is usually dull and ill-defined, like June's was. Bleeding and weight loss can also occur. Colon cancer on the left side, or in the sigmoid area, manifests more often in changes in bowel habits, an increased use of laxatives, bleeding, gas pain, constipation, or narrowing of the stool.

16

Most colon cancer symptoms—despite a similarity to other conditions—fall into the following four areas.

1. **Obstruction.** Colon cancers commonly grow, and the tumor becomes larger than the inner passageway—or lumen. The colonic lumen is widest in the cecum and ascending colon on the right side of the abdomen, and obstruction is much less likely to occur there. However, in the transverse colon, which crosses the abdomen near the navel, and in the descending and sigmoid colons, on the left side of the abdomen, the passageway is narrower, and, thus, obstruction is more likely to occur. If the colonic lumen is completely blocked, pressure builds and causes pain and swelling of the abdomen. Nausea and vomiting might occur if the obstruction is extreme.

2. **Bleeding.** As tumors expand into the passageway, they are traumatized by the fecal stream, and this causes them to bleed. If the tumor is near the anus, the blood might be visible. But it is much more common for the blood to be hidden in stool. If such bleeding continues for months, it can cause iron deficiency anemia, evidence of which is sought, therefore, in making a diagnosis. But although bleeding is the most common symptom of colon cancer, only 20 percent of patients with rectal bleeding have colon cancer. Bleeding can mean any number of things, including hemorrhoids.

3. **Pain.** When invasive cells from the tumor eventually penetrate the wall of the colon and invade adjacent tissue, pain is felt, and other specific symptoms, depending on the organ invaded, appear. For example, if cancer cells penetrate into the bladder, urinary symptoms might appear. Sometimes physicians are drawn to the liver or bone because of a patient's pain and only later find a primary tumor in the colon, where it has produced hardly any symptoms at all.

4. **A Wasting Syndrome.** Some tumors cause loss of appetite, weight, and strength. This can be all out of proportion to the size of the tumor.

So, there is much to investigate. The good news is that today, doctors have much better diagnostic tools than they did years ago—they can view the entire digestive system with sophisticated endoscopic equipment and easily take tissue samples for biopsy, to more efficiently determine if there is cancer present.

In the next chapter, the screening process will be explained.

2

GUIDELINES FOR ACCURATE DIAGNOSIS

Colon cancer is preventable and curable through early detection, but less than half the population gets the screening needed for early detection, and thus for cure. This could probably be blamed on the failure of health insurers to pay for such screening or on the unpleasantness associated with an invasive procedure. But in truth, there is simply not enough public awareness about the importance of early detection in preventing colon cancer.

Endoscopic screening procedures are not nearly as unpleasant as most people think. Endoscopes are flexible tubes containing tiny video cameras that are inserted into the body through the oral or rectal cavity. A camera allows close inspection of the digestive system. A flexible sigmoidoscopy, for instance, takes from 5 to 10 minutes in the doctor's office and causes about as much discomfort as a mild gas pain. The trip through the colon appears on the video monitor so the patient and the physician can watch. Still pictures from the video monitor are kept in a patient's file so they can be studied again and again by both the patient and the treatment team. A patient can also get copies of these pictures.

The American Cancer Society, The National Cancer Institute, the American College of Surgeons, and the American College of Physicians all recommend that average-risk people begin screening for colon cancer at age 50 with annual sigmoidoscopies, preferably flexible endoscopic sigmoidoscopies, every three to five years. The American Cancer Society and the National Cancer Institute also recommend an annual digital rectal examination for everyone over

50, but there is some controversy about whether this is helpful. The value of fecal occult blood testing for screening remains even more controversial.

Examining the colon and rectum of asymptomatic adults as a means of detecting colon and rectal cancers and polyps has been the subject of several studies and a good deal of controversy. In one investigation, total colonoscopy was performed in 209 average-risk adults, 50 to 75 years of age, who had no symptoms and who tested negative for the presence of occult blood in the stool. Two people of this group were discovered to have colon or rectal cancers, and as many as half had polyps. All of the polyps were larger than 1 centimeter. Both cancers occurred in people over the age of 60. Half of the people with adenomas and one of those with colon cancer showed no findings beyond the reach of the flexible fiberoptic sigmoidoscope.

The average person over 50 has a 5 to 6 percent chance of developing colon cancer by the age of 80 and a 2.5 percent chance of dying from it. And if a first-degree relative—parent, sibling, or child—under 55 had colon cancer, screening should begin at age 40. This standard of care is not yet in full use because most medical insurance does not cover the cost. One of the most urgent medical issues today is convincing Medicare, Medicaid, and other health insurers that preventive screening for colon cancer is imperative in order to save lives. It costs much more to treat colon cancer than to prevent it.

Because the symptoms of colon cancer are so nonspecific—gaseousness, abdominal discomfort and pain, a change in bowel-habit pattern—many colon and rectal cancers have time to grow, to invade the wall of the colon, and to spread to regional lymph nodes and sometimes other vital body organs before they come to medical attention. With regular screening, all colon cancer would be discovered and treated before it became fatal. Tests available for colon cancer screening include digital rectal examination, fecal occult blood testing, sigmoidoscopy (preferably fiberoptic), colonoscopy, and barium enema X ray.

Even if you get regular annual physical checkup, it is not enough, without the specific screenings for colon cancer. Physical examination, such as digital exam by itself or palpating the abdomen, often do not detect signs of colon or rectal malignancy.

Stool testing for occult blood and laboratory examinations such as blood count to detect anemia, iron levels, and liver blood tests provide some additional information. But the only sure way to find and identify polyps in the colon and rectum is with the barium enema X ray; the flexible fiberoptic sigmoidoscopy, which examines the lower third of the colon and rectum; and colonoscopy, which examines the entire colon.

DIGITAL RECTAL EXAMINATION (DRE)

A DRE should be part of everyone's annual physical examination beginning at the age of 40. The American Cancer Society and the National Cancer Institute believe this test is effective as a screening tool for colon cancer for everyone over the age of 50. (However, arguments for this in the medical community are not strongly substantiated.) With this simple examination, the physician is able to explore the lower part of the rectum for polyps.

The rectum is the final extension of the sigmoid colon and is about 5 inches long. When the patient bears down during the examination, he or she is able to bring down more of the lower rectum and sigmoid colon for examination. About 20 percent of colon cancers develop in the rectum, and these tumors are detected by DRE in 75 percent of cases. An infiltrating cancer feels hard and irregular, whereas a benign polyp is more likely to be soft and pliable. About 10 percent of cancers occurring in the rectum can be detected this way.

FECAL OCCULT BLOOD TEST (FOBT)

Because the loss of blood that is hidden in the stool is the most common sign of cancer of the colon and rectum, fecal occult blood test, first introduced to clinical practice in the 1950s, has come to be regarded as a valuable aid in colorectal and gastrointestinal cancer surveillance. A 13-year study of 46,000 patients at the University of Minnesota resulted in a 33 percent reduction of cancer mortality by screening with an annual FOBT. But keep in mind that many benign conditions cause this bleeding, too.

The FOBT is a simple test using a card on which samples of stool can be smeared and analyzed. The currently available guaiac-impregnated cards are very accurate when used properly. These cards are most often given to patients by their physicians, but FOBT cards are often available at hospital and health fairs (such as those in communities or malls), and from nurses or health offices in the workplace. And, like the home pregnancy tests, the FOBT kits are also available over the counter in some drug stores.

The collection of two smears per day from different parts of the stool for three days is recommended. A chemical is applied to the samples at the doctor's office or at a laboratory, or a person can do it at home. If the sample turns blue, it indicates the presence of blood in the stool.

The fecal occult blood test is far from a perfect method for screening for colorectal cancer, but it is constantly undergoing refinements. It is recommended by the American Cancer Society to complement more invasive procedures for the detection of colon cancer. Annual fecal occult blood testing has been shown to significantly decrease the cumulative mortality from colorectal cancer when performed regularly to the general population for more than a decade.

In a large clinical trial still in progress at Memorial Sloan-Kettering Medical Center in New York City, only 38.5 percent of patients offered the free screening returned their cards. Of those, 4.1 percent had a positive test, and of those who tested positive, 36 percent were found to have colon cancer. The study clearly indicates that a substantial number of cancers can be detected in their early stage with FOBT.

Before testing for hidden blood, patients are often asked to follow a special diet for two days because the digestion of certain foods can cause a false positive or false negative result. (Patients do not always comply with these dietary restrictions, and some do not follow the number of samples required.) For example, fiber is allowed because it is believed to stimulate bleeding from any existing polyps protruding into the colon passageway. On the other hand, aspirin is to be avoided because it can cause bleeding that has nothing to do with a possible polyp in the colon and it could cause a false positive result.

Other foods and substances to avoid for that reason include red meat, turnips, horseradish, citrus fruits and vitamin C, and iron supplements. Patients are asked to eat high-fiber foods, such as bran, peanuts, and popcorn, as well as fruits and vegetables, chicken, and tuna fish.

FLEXIBLE SIGMOIDOSCOPY

There has been a significant reduction in colon cancer deaths because of the increase in diagnostic-screening sigmoidoscopy. Even one screening in a 10-year period reduced the risk by 79 percent according to a study at the University of Wisconsin. Approximately two-thirds of colon polyps are within reach of the flexible fiberoptic proctosigmoidoscope. This instrument—about 1.5 to 2 feet long—sends a tiny video camera into the sigmoid area, or left side of the colon. This instrument is widely used today, replacing the more objectionable rigid instruments in use until the 1970s. This older technique is far from ideal for screening purposes. It is unpopular with patients and physicians and provides consistent examination of only the lower 16 centimeters—about 6.25 inches—of the colon and rectum.

If you are preparing for a flexible sigmoidoscopy, which can be done in your gastroenterologist's office or the endoscopy suite of a hospital, your doctor might have you self-administer two enemas at home the night before. (An *enema* is the insertion of fluid into the rectum through the anus, which causes the evacuation of fecal matter from the rectum.) Some doctors prescribe a gentle overnight laxative preparation. You will be asked to refrain from eating after midnight and to come to the procedure with an empty colon. No sedation is necessary for this procedure, but you might occasionally feel some pressure, like a gas pain.

While you lie on your side, the endoscopist manipulates the scope through your colon. If you are curious, you can watch the progress of the scope on the video monitor with your physician. The colon is flexible, with many loops and folds, and appears pink on the video monitor.

When a polyp is found during a sigmoidoscopy, it is customary to recommend colonoscopy so the entire colon can be inspected. It is mandatory to see the rest of the colon because of the chance that there are more polyps farther up in the colon. Then, the initial polyp and any others can be removed and biopsied at the same time. It is standard practice to remove all polyps at the time of detection with colonoscopy, and it would be unethical to leave polyps in place for observation. (See Chapter 6 for a review of the polypectomy procedure.)

BARIUM ENEMA X RAY

This X-ray procedure is sometimes used in conjunction with sigmoidoscopy to provide complementary information, especially if an obstruction is detected. The barium enema X ray is still a time-honored tool for finding polyps, but not all physicians find it necessary. Most believe that if a polyp is found with sigmoid-oscopy, then the patient should proceed to the more accurate colonoscopy to examine the entire length of the colon and should have the polyp removed and biopsied at the same time. However, some health insurance companies and health maintenance organizations might require the barium enema X ray as part of the screening procedure for colon cancer because it is generally less expensive than colonoscopy.

If this is the case with your health insurance coverage, talk with your physician. You might be able to ask the insurance company to make an exception, or you might be able to pay for the procedure at a reduced rate.

After the colon is cleansed with enemas, an inert substance containing barium is inserted into the rectum and colon through the anus. Barium appears opaque on X rays. The camera watches under fluoroscopic guidance and X-ray pictures as the barium fills the colon and rectum. To make small tumors easier to see, the doctor might also expand the colon by carefully pumping in air during the test. This is called an air contrast or double-contrast barium enema and improves the accuracy of the standard barium enema X ray.

A technician generally performs a large part of the procedure in conjunction with a physician (radiologist). The physician will look at the films as they are developed and possibly again later on. The sensitivity of this screening procedure is directly related to the patience and diligence of the technician and physician performing the procedure. Overlapping loops of bowel can be difficult to interpret, and extensive diverticulosis or residual fecal material can also interfere with an accurate reading. There is normally a small risk associated with radiation exposure, but the real limitation in this procedure is that a biopsy or polypectomy cannot be performed if a polyp is discovered.

COLONOSCOPY

Colonoscopy is the most accurate and preferred diagnostic tool for seeing the entire colon up to 95 percent of the time. Many studies have shown that a colonoscopy detects polyps often left undetected by a barium enema X ray. Also, a physician and a technician perform this procedure simultaneously, so there are two pairs of experienced eyes searching the inside of the colon. Colonoscopy has the highest diagnostic sensitivity and allows a polypectomy—removal of the polyp—to be done at the same time if necessary.

The colonoscope is a fiberoptic tube about the width of your smallest finger and as long as the colon, up to six feet. Additional instruments can be inserted through this tube, such as a snare or wire loop to sever a polyp with an electrical current. Forceps can be passed through it to remove a piece of tissue from the colon lining for biopsy. A small brush can collect epithelial cells for study under the microscope. A patient could have a small cancer in the cecum, and when it is discovered with colonoscopy and removed right then, the survival rate is high—85 to 90 percent. Colonoscopy is generally an outpatient procedure performed in a doctor's office or an endoscopy suite at a hospital.

- **Before a colonoscopy.** For a colonoscopy to be effective, the colon must be absolutely clean of fecal matter. This flushing out is done with enemas, with traditional laxatives, or with a nonabsorbable lavage solution that you drink ahead of time. The oral lavage solution passes through the intestines instead of being absorbed into the urine and causes a liquid stool. There are six or seven different types of oral lavage available, and most come in flavors—cherry or pineapple—to make them more palatable; but they still taste like salty or soapy water. Your doctor will tell you which one to buy at your drug store. These lavage solutions come in powdered form in a one-gallon plastic jug that you simply fill with water. You will need to prepare the solution the day before your exam, according to instructions on the package. Store this in your refrigerator and then have a regular breakfast. Your fasting will begin with lunch, which can be a light liquid, such as soup or broth, and perhaps a gelatin dessert—but it should not be red gelatin because it could mimic the appearance of blood.

Then, between 5 P.M. and 6 P.M., you will begin drinking the lavage solution, usually an eight-ounce glass every 10 to 15 minutes for about three hours. Prepare to spend the evening near the bathroom because the lavage will flush out your system quickly. It is important to drink an entire glassful every 10 or 15 minutes. If you sip small amounts all during the evening, it will not work as well. Remember, unless your colon is completely cleaned and flushed out, the colonoscopy will not be effective. Poor results could mean you will have to do it again.

If you are at home, you might want to pace yourself with a timer. In the hospital, a family member or friend can help you keep track of the intervals. You have three hours to consume all of the lavage. By approximately 9 P.M. you should be finished with the last of the lavage solution, and by 10 P.M. you should have completely emptied your colon, although you might feel bloated or gassy. Get a good night's rest.

Never hesitate to call your doctor if you have any questions or problems with drinking the lavage and getting ready for your colonoscopy. Physicians always expect some phone calls the night before a procedure. Some patients call to ask if they can take the lavage after taking their other medications. Some might complain of chills or vomiting necessitating the physician's attention.

The morning of the colonoscopy, you can have eight ounces of clear liquid, such as coffee or tea, clear juice, soup, or water. *But don't drink anything within an hour of your exam.*

Your physician will need to know about medications you are taking. Aspirin products, arthritis medications, blood thinners, insulin, and iron supplements might be suspended for a period. If you have ever needed antibiotics during dental procedures, let your doctor know. You might need them for a colonoscopy as well to kill any bacteria that might become dislodged during the procedure and invade heart valves, for example.

- **The procedure.** Before the procedure begins, you might be given an intravenous (IV) narcotic analgesic (pain killer) such as Demerol®. An IV sedation such as Valium® or Versed® might be used to induce a state of "conscious sedation" so that you are relaxed. A respiratory monitor—a device called a pulse-oximeter—will be clipped on to the end of your finger to measure your pulse and oxygen-saturation level during the procedure. Your blood pressure will also be monitored.

Expect your physician to talk with you about any past experience you had with this kind of screening. Your doctor wants you to be comfortable and not apprehensive, and it is reassuring if you have a dialogue with him or her. A caring physician is of utmost importance for the success of this procedure.

Remember, your colon is a tube as long as 5 feet full of turns and bends, so the trip through it might take from 15 minutes to an hour. Because you have been sedated, you should not feel any severe discomfort, except for a bit of gaseousness or an urge to move your bowels. The colon, by the way, cannot sense many things that would cause pain, only distension and tugging. You will be lying on your side or your back most of the time while the colonoscope is advancing into your colon, but you might be asked to change position from time to time in order to move the colonoscope around for better viewing. The colon lining is studied once again while the colonoscope is slowly withdrawn. This procedure is accurate if the patient is well prepared and the physician skilled at moving the endoscope around.

After the colonoscopy, you will feel fine, but because you have been sedated, you must rest for as long as two hours before you can go home. And somebody must take you home. You will not be allowed to leave on your own, drive a car, or operate machinery.

• **After a colonoscopy.** You might feel some abdominal discomfort or distension for several hours after the procedure. Because there is air in your abdominal cavity and diaphragm, you might also have the hiccups, feel bloated, or have some cramps caused by the air in your colon. This should disappear quickly with the passage of gas. Unless a polyp was removed, you should be able to resume normal eating and activity after you leave.

Although colonoscopy is a very invasive examination, complications are rare. Most dreaded is perforation of the colon with the colonoscope, but this is extremely rare. Less serious and more common is hemorrhaging after removal of a polyp or a piece of tissue for biopsy. If you believe something is wrong or if you have a fever and chills, rectal bleeding, or severe abdominal pain after a colonoscopy, call your physician immediately.

(See Chapter 6 for more information about polypectomy.)

OTHER IMAGING TECHNIQUES

Occasionally, a finding seen on endoscopic examination cannot be identified, or there is need to further investigate a mass or density in the wall of the colon, such as inflamed diverticula. Then, other techniques for seeing into this section of your colon might be used.

Endoscopic Ultrasound

Ultrasound is sometimes used to supplement endoscopy to determine if a lesion is solid. The physician or technician scans the colon with a colonoscope monitored outside your abdomen by a handheld transducer or probe that converts the sound waves that bounce off your body into images on a screen.

CAT (or CT) Scan

Because your surgeon will be able to look at and feel your liver and other organs when he or she begins open abdominal surgery, a computerized axial tomography (CAT) scan is not always considered necessary. However, a CAT scan is an excellent way to look at your abdominal wall and the lymph-node-bearing areas of your abdomen, liver, and other solid organs for signs of metastasis. While you lie inside a wide tube, this X ray translates information into two dimensional "slices," or cross sections. The radiation dose from a CAT scan is considerably higher than a routine X ray. The amount depends on the number of slices needed and on the part of the body. A CAT scan is also used in planning radiation treatment to outline the field or area to be treated.

Magnetic Resonance Imaging (MRI)

MRI is not generally used to screen for colon cancer because it is costly and less specific than colonoscopy, sigmoidoscopy, or barium enema X ray. Like a CAT scan, it can give a better image of the solid abdominal organs and lymph nodes than that obtained by the other methods. Scientists are developing the MRI capability to differentiate between malignant and benign processes and to evaluate lymph nodes for metastasis. Patients are often afraid of the procedure because it means being confined in a long tube for as long as an hour. However, a mild sedative makes most claustrophobic patients relax. At some diagnostic centers, open-air MRI is becoming available.

CHOOSING A GASTROENTEROLOGIST, ENDOSCOPIST, OR SCREENING CENTER

Most people have no experience with endoscopic diagnostic procedures until they need them. Suppose your family doctor finds a suspicious lesion while performing a digital rectal exam. This means you need to have a sigmoidoscopy or colonoscopy. In talking with your family, it turns out Uncle Harry had one of those done years ago and says any doctor can do it. Why bother with the time and expense of a specialist?

Most primary-care physicians are not trained in the use of endoscopic procedures and will refer you to a gastroenterologist or surgeon specially trained in this procedure. So, although Uncle Harry might be wise in many ways, it would be better in this case to ask your family doctor to recommend a gastroenterologist or a medical center that can do gastroenterological screenings—flexible sigmoidoscopy or colonoscopy.

Endoscopy Defined

As part of their education, gastroenterologists receive extensive endoscopic training in performing colonoscopy, polypectomy, and biopsy thoroughly, safely, and with a minimum amount of patient discomfort. Some surgeons also receive this training, particularly if they are subspecialists known as colorectal surgeons.

Endoscopic sigmoidoscopy can be done without a video monitor. The physician peers through the endoscope and searches the inside of the colon. He or she is the only one who sees what is there, and there are often no permanent pictures for you to take with you or for physicians to consult for further study.

Find out if there is video equipment for the procedure or if the doctor will be viewing by eyeball through the endoscopic tube. Most major medical centers and most gastroenterologists will have state-of-the-art endoscopic equipment with video. This provides much better visual view of the colon and makes diagnosis much more effective. And it provides better documentation. You will have pictures you can carry with you to other members of your treatment team and to second or third opinions.

Questions to Ask

There are certain standards for endoscopic procedures recognized by the American Society of Gastrointestinal Endoscopy that can help you make your choice. Before you consent to having an endoscopic procedure done, ask the following questions.

- Where did the physician receive his or her training in endoscopy? A gastroenterologist is trained in endoscopy by other physicians as part of his or her postgraduate medical training. Ask about the doctor's training before you get ready for the procedure, not the minute before the colonoscope is to be inserted into your body.

- Will the procedure be monitored by video? This is the best procedure, and you can retain hard copy pictures of the procedure, as well.

- Do the physicians and technicians performing endoscopic procedures observe universal precautions? They should abide by these precautions, which means they wear gloves, masks, and gowns during the procedure.

- Will anything be removed, such as a polyp or a piece of tissue?

- Will a biopsy be done? A biopsy is standard practice whenever a polyp or a piece of tissue is removed from the colon.

- Where and by whom will the biopsy be examined? Ask about the pathologist and the pathology laboratory. Find out if the pathology will be done in the same medical center or sent out to another laboratory. You might check this with your insurance company, as well, to make sure they cover the particular pathology lab.

- Will the pathologist come in during the procedure to also watch the video monitor before taking any tissue or polyp samples back to the lab?

- How long will it take for the pathology report? For the procedure report? It will usually take about four business days to find out the results. Ask for an estimated time to call for results. Understand that if this takes longer, it does not necessarily mean the results are bad; it only means your anxiety level is higher. Sometimes there are delays in hospitals and labs.

- Will you be given conscious sedation with medications such as Demerol®, Valium®, or Versed®? And who will give you the anesthesia if it is used? Sometimes an anesthetist is require to administer these substances, and sometimes the gastroenterolo-

31

gist can do it. This depends on the regulations of the particular diagnostic center.

- Find out the plans for going home following your colonoscopy or sigmoidoscopy and what diet should be followed.
- Who will be present during the procedure? Generally, a gastroenterologist does the procedure with the help of an assistant who may be a technician or a physician's assistant or nurse.
- What will it cost and what does the cost include?

To find a medical center with proper endoscopic standards in your area, you can also call one of the cancer information hotlines listed in Appendix 1, or check local health networks. Sometimes the human resources department where you work can be helpful. They are often aware of employee and corporate health plans that include low-cost screenings.

THE COST OF SCREENING

Some of the routine costs of screening, such as the DRE and the FOBT, are minimal. These are normally included as part of routine physical examinations.

Endoscopic sigmoidoscopy costs approximately $50 to $250. Not all insurance carriers cover this cost, but Medicare now covers part of the cost if it is for screening purposes. The cost of a barium enema X ray ranges from $200 to $500 and is commonly covered, at least in part, by most health insurers.

The cost of colonoscopy has come down a bit in recent years and is usually in a range of between $300 and $1,200. Keep in mind that the procedure itself is only part of the cost; so, before you have the procedure, ask what the cost covers. You do not want to be surprised later to find out about a room-use fee of $1,000. There might also be such charges as a professional fee, a room fee, and tray charges and charges for nursing, medications, the preparation, biopsy, pathology, and polypectomy. These are just some of the charges you can encounter, so be sure to ask your doctor for all this information. Call your insurance company as well to be sure you know what is covered. A colonoscopy is often not covered by medical insurance if it is for screening purposes. However, Medicare now covers more of the cost than it did in the past.

THE FUTURE: VIRTUAL COLONOSCOPY

Virtual colonoscopy, an examination of the colon without an invasive tube, has been in experimental stage for some time at Wake Forest University in North Carolina and at other research centers and might possibly lead to less invasive diagnostic techniques. Virtual colonoscopy combines X rays and computers to view inside the entire colon without inserting anything but air. This is a relatively new form of X-ray technology called *spiral CAT*. The exam would take 30 seconds and requires no sedation. It would cost half as much as a colonoscopy.

One day, people might be able to predict their overall susceptibility to colon cancer with a quick rectal biopsy in the doctor's office. Such a test would survey the proliferation of epithelial cells of the colon, one of the earliest findings in patients with ulcerative colitis, a known risk factor for colon cancer. The same proliferation is found in familial adenomatous polyposis (FAP) patients and sporadic colon cancer families. If such a defect exists, a sample of the rectal mucosa could be valuable in estimating cancer risk, similar to the way the Pap smear can detect the risk of ovarian cancer.

Ongoing research in molecular biology and genetics is seeking to identify markers of colon cancer risk that might someday allow for total prevention. Researchers are studying certain mutations in the colons of people with curable colon cancer, looking for other biomarkers of early detection. Both fatty acids and bile salts, thought to be implicated in colon cancer, are under investigation.

Someday, people will be able to use a simple blood test to detect colon cancer. But until then, diagnostic screening for early detection is the *only* prevention.

3

BIOPSY AND STAGING

The *pathologist,* a physician who specializes in the microscopic study (histology) of human tissue, is a very important part of the treatment team for colon cancer. There is much to be learned from the study of a polyp or tissue from the colon lining, and this information is critical to diagnosis and treatment. The pathologist might come to the endoscopic suite during a colonoscopy and polypectomy to discuss with the gastroenterologist the preparations for biopsy. These two physicians work together in interpreting their findings and staging the cancer.

If the pathologist discovers cancer in a polyp or in the cells of the colon or rectal mucosa, then the most important determination to be made will be whether the cancer has penetrated the colon lining and wall. And if the cancer is invasive—meaning it has broken through the colon wall or has the potential to do so—then a surgical biopsy of lymph nodes and a section of the colon might be necessary because it gives the doctors a chance to get the most information microscopically about what is going on. And they can also look at the cancer and surrounding tissue with their own eyes. This is called gross examination.

WHAT TO KNOW BEFORE AN ENDOSCOPIC BIOPSY

For purposes of biopsy, part or all of a polyp can be removed or a piece of the colon lining can be removed. One of the benefits of colonoscopy is that the polyp can be removed when it is discovered in a low-risk procedure. The pedunculated polyp has a stalk and is easily removed at the base with a wire snare through which an electric current is passed, permitting the polyp to be cauterized. The sessile polyp, on the other hand, has no stalk, and sometimes it cannot be completely removed either because it is not raised from the mucosa or because it is too small. When encountered, sessile polyps should be extensively biopsied or "shaved" with the resulting fragments recovered and sent to the pathologist.

Only a small percentage of polyps show cancer, but all colonic polyps must be distinguished from carcinomas, and complete biopsies are critical. If a polyp is too large—bigger than 3 or 4 centimeters (about 1.5 inches), only a piece of it might be removed. A 2-centimeter polyp that is flat cannot always be removed as easily as a pedunculated polyp that is attached to the colon wall by a stalk.

It is important to know what kind of polyp was removed and if it was completely or only partially removed. Partial biopsy could be misleading. If one piece of polyp is okay, there could still be cancer cells in the other part of the polyp. Ask your physician about this.

Also, if a polyp with a stalk is removed and part of the stalk remains attached to the colon lining, another biopsy might be needed if cancer was found in the polyp. It is important to be sure no cancer has escaped into the remaining stalk. However, there are many "ifs" for patient and doctor to consider. Some medical literature claims removal of a polyp is enough. But some patients and doctors might ask about whether the stalk was cut straight. What if invasive cancer cells have passed through that stalk into the lining? This is why it is so important for patients to review the pathology findings, to discuss these findings thoughtfully with their physicians, and to get a second opinion if necessary, possibly from a colorectal surgeon.

Whether a patient is undergoing a biopsy or removal of a polyp, the colon must be properly cleansed, and blood tests must be done in advance to ascertain the platelet count and how the blood coagulates. This is especially important if a patient has a history of bleeding, such as a blood-clotting disorder like hemophilia. Special precautions and additional work is needed if a patient takes a blood thinner such as Coumadin®. Many physicians insist that the patient forego the use of aspirin and nonsteroidal anti-inflammatory drugs for a week to 10 days before biopsy or polyp removal and for several days after the biopsy because of the effects these medications can have on the blood-coagulation process. This is to minimize the risk of hemorrhage.

An extremely rare complication of removing a polyp is hemorrhage from the vessel that supplies blood to the body of the polyp. Another possible complication is perforation—formation of a hole—in the wall of the colon. The removal of large sessile polyps, as opposed to small- to moderate-sized pedunculated polyps is more likely to predispose the patient to these complications.

UNDER THE MICROSCOPE

When the pathologist studies the colonic tissue under the microscope, many things are revealed. The tumor size is measured. The edges of the polyp are checked to see if the tumor extends to those edges, or "margins." The most important job for the pathologist is to determine the depth of invasion, but a thorough analysis of the polyp or colonic tissue requires many studies.

The tumor cells are examined to determine if they are invasive, how fast they are growing, and how aggressive they are. If the cancer is invasive, further tests might be done. These pieces of information—the variables of colon cancer—are called *prognostic indicators*. They help guide both patient and doctors with decision making about treatment. For example, approximately 20 percent of colon carcinomas are poorly differentiated or undifferentiated tumors. This means the cells are aggressive and likely to invade other organs. Most carcinomas secrete a small or moderate amount of mucin, but about 10 to 20 percent of tumors are described as *mucinous* or *colloid carcinomas* because they produce *large* amounts of mucin. Mucinous carcinomas are also more aggressive. The grade of a cancer labels the overall pattern of the tumor cells and nuclei. It also tells how aggressive the cancer is. If it is Grade 1, then it is the least aggressive form. Grade 3 is the most aggressive and the most common.

The College of American Pathologists has developed a standard of guidelines and protocol for the histologic study of colorectal carcinoma—for both local excision (polypectomy) and surgical resection (colectomy). This also includes guidelines about the particular information the pathologist must receive from the other physicians in order to perform his or her task accurately.

Some of the things a patient should expect to see in a pathology report include depth of invasion, type and grade of the carcinoma, and evidence of vascular invasion or invasion of the stalk or submucosa. A biopsy after abdominal surgery to remove the diseased piece of colon should also include the status of the margins on a resected piece of colon and presence or absence of cancer cells in the lymph nodes.

THE SURGICAL BIOPSY

Once it has been determined that cancer has invaded the colon wall, more pathological examinations will be done after surgery.

- **Colon section.** The section of the colon that is removed during surgery is sent to the lab, where it is measured and tested for a number of indicators. As a matter of routine, the pathologist will look to see if the tumor involved the "edges" of what the surgeon has removed. If so, that generally means cancer has spread. Distal and proximal margins are anatomical locations on the piece of colon resected. *Distal* is toward the rectum, and *proximal* is toward the cecum. Generally, the only time the proximal and distal margins are both positive for cancer is when the disease is low lying in the colon, near the rectum and sphincter muscle. In that tightly congested area, it is not possible to remove a large enough section of colon to allow for clean margins. Then, removal of the rectum and a colostomy is usually necessary.
- **Lymph nodes.** Some lymph nodes around the colon section will also be removed for study. These lymph nodes are usually found in the mesenteric layer of fat around the colon and are early indicators of whether or not cancer has spread from the colon. These nodes are a critical prognostic factor of a patient's diagnosis. Are they negative or positive for cancer? The number of lymph nodes analyzed depends on the size of the piece of colon removed.

Lymph nodes are glands that act as the filters in the body's drainage system, and they are encased in fatty tissue in strategic locations throughout the body. The lymphatic fluid flows away from the colon through the mesentery. Each person has different sizes, shapes, and patterns of lymph nodes. Some have heavy clusters of nodes like bunches of grapes. Others have nodes spread out and far apart like marbles dropped on the floor. Some nodes are as small as sesame seeds, others as big as jelly beans. Sometimes they are enlarged from infection or inflammation or if they are filled with cancer cells.

It is possible to have a large colon cancer tumor and no affected lymph nodes. Each case must be treated individually. If the cancer has spread to the lymph nodes, it means there is an increased risk for systemic recurrence of colon cancer. Any lymph node showing cancer is evaluated to see if the cancer is contained inside the node or has broken through the shell of the node. A pathologist might examine, on average, about 10 lymph nodes. For some reason, there are usually more lymph nodes around the right colon, the cecum, and fewer on the left side, around the sigmoid colon. Lymph node status, along with tumor size, is one of the most important prognostic indicators, crucial to treatment planning. With even one lymph node showing cancer, a patient should talk with a medical oncologist about the risk of systemic and local recurrence of colon cancer and whether chemotherapy is needed.

INTERPRETING YOUR PATHOLOGY REPORTS

Surprisingly, few patients ask to see their pathology reports. These written reports are sent by the pathologist to the gastroenterologist or surgeon, who tells the patient what it says and puts it in his or her file. You can ask for your own copy of the report so you can ask questions about what it contains. This report gives you information that you need to understand treatment, and you should become familiar with it. For example, the study of the cells in your tumor can affect choices or dosages of medications to use in chemotherapy. Ask your gastroenterologist, surgeon, or oncologist to tell you what everything means in these reports, and how they (the doctors) interpret the report. Take it with you if you talk with other doctors for additional opinions.

The first biopsy report will tell you about your polyp or tumor, and subsequent operative reports will evaluate your lymph nodes and a colon section. It should take no more than seven days from the time of biopsy until receipt of the report. Doctors often hear a preliminary report from the pathologist by phone, so you might have some information sooner.

Here is a typical report from a surgical biopsy of a colon section and lymph nodes. These findings led doctors to the decision that the patient's prognosis was good and that no further treatment was needed.

A centrally ulcerating peripherally fungating tumor which extends above the mucosa. On cross section, the tumor invaded into but not through the colon wall. A section of the mesentery was removed so lymph nodes could be measured and tested. All 17 nodes were negative. The surgical margins were free of tumor, and the cells were moderately differentiated.

This report meant that the polyp was ulcerated, so it was probably bleeding. Further investigation showed that the cancer cells were not particularly aggressive and that no cancer had yet traveled to the lymph nodes, so chances were good that the cancer did not spread.

Another pathologist's report for a colon section from a 65-year-old man showed a much larger tumor in the cecum, with cells moderately to poorly differentiating, and the tumor invaded through the colon wall. Although there was no vascular invasion or perineural invasion of the connective tissue around the nerves, the cancer had traveled to the lymph nodes. Five of 11 lymph nodes tested contained metastatic cancer cells. This diagnosis as advanced colon cancer called for aggressive systemic treatment.

HOW COLON CANCER IS STAGED

Once your biopsies—endoscopic and surgical—have been completed, your cancer can be "staged." This is a rather elaborate

39

classification system based on the sum of many variables. Everything your doctors have learned about your colon cancer, from its physical appearance through all the tests, are classified and subclassified: size, type, location of tumor, depth of invasion, cell activity. Stage is generally the most important prognostic indicator.

Duke's Classification

The stage of the colon cancer and your general health help determine your treatment options. A system called Modified Duke's Classification is the most widely used to stage colon cancer.

- Duke's Stage A is cancer in situ, or high-grade dysplasia and means cancer is limited to the mucous membrane that lines the colon (mucosa or submucosa). Five-year-survival rate after treatment is 90 percent.
- Duke's Stage B1 means cancer has penetrated into but not through the *muscularis propria,* a deeper layer of the colon wall. Five-year-survival rate after treatment is 80 percent.
- Duke's Stage B2 means cancer has penetrated through the *muscularis propria* or the *serosa,* the outer lining of the colon wall. Five-year-survival rate is 70 percent.
- Duke's Stage C1 is the same as B1 plus lymph node metastases. Five-year-survival rate after treatment is 50 percent.
- Duke's Stage C2 is same as B2 plus lymph node involvement. Five-year-survival rate is 50 percent.
- Duke's Stage D means there is distant metastases. Survival rate after treatment is generally less than five years.

The TNM System

Another system physicians use to provide uniform pathologic categories is the TNM System—tumor, nodes, metastasis.

- **Tumor**
  Tis—carcinoma in situ.
  T1 indicates submucosal invasion (Duke's Stage A).

T2 indicates invasion of the *muscularis propria* (Duke's Stage B1).

T3 indicates invasion through the *muscularis propria* into the subserosa or perirectal tissues (Duke's Stage B2).

T4 indicates invasion into adjacent organs or tissues (Duke's Stage B3).

- **Nodes**

  N0—no involved lymph nodes.

  N1—one to three regional lymph node metastases (Duke's Stage C1).

  N2—more than three regional lymph node metastases (Duke's Stage C2).

  N3—a metastasis along the course of a major blood vessel.

- **Metastasis**

  M0—no distant metastases.

  M1—metastases present.

The grade or stage of the cancer is also a significant influence in prognosis. For example, patients whose cancers are Grades 1 and 2 have better five-year-survival rates than those with Grade 3. The location of the tumor is an independent factor. Among patients with the same stage disease, rectal carcinomas might be more difficult to cure than carcinomas in the colon. And in the colon itself, transverse and descending colon carcinomas seem to result in poorer outcomes than those in the ascending or sigmoid colon.

Ask your physician how he or she arrived at your particular staging. Although there are precise and standard guidelines, there are always situations that might fall between two categories, so it is sometimes a judgment call on the part of the physicians.

SOME HEALTH INSURANCE CONSIDERATIONS ABOUT BIOPSY

Most medical insurance covers the cost of biopsy procedures, laboratory tests, and pathology fees, but not always all of them. Health maintenance organizations (HMOs) often require that biopsies be done only by certain laboratories with whom they have contracts, and the place your doctor has chosen to have your pathology study done might not be one of them.

Tests will cost several hundred dollars, so check to be sure that the particular pathology lab accepts your medical insurance. If not, discuss this with your surgeon and find out what other alternatives you have. You might be able to negotiate a reduced charge if your surgeon prefers to use that particular lab. It is not uncommon for your surgeon to be part of your medical plan coverage, but not the laboratory, even if they operate in the same medical center.

Why You Must Be Well Informed

Suppose you have an endoscopic examination in your doctor's office, and a polyp is removed, but the hospital's pathology fee is not covered by your insurance. Your insurer will only pay for pathology done by an outside commercial lab. However, if you are in a comprehensive cancer center, your surgeon will not be able to make a surgical decision based on an outside commercial laboratory biopsy. He or she will want one done in the same place where the screening was done. Outside commercial laboratories are often acceptable to doctors for analysis of potassium levels and other blood tests but not for anything as critical as a tissue biopsy. If your biopsy was done at an outside commercial lab, your surgeon must get the biopsy slides from another laboratory or hospital and then have them analyzed again by his or her hospital pathology staff. This will double the cost of biopsy, and the insurance will likely not cover it.

Doctors are used to working with other doctors they know as part of a "multidisciplinary" team to treat a patient. Mutual trust, a common hospital, complementary training, and professional competence are a part of the "glue" holding together these teams. Current trends in health insurance do not necessarily recognize these groups, and the teams might be fragmented if one or more physicians necessary to your care are not covered in your plan. This sometimes results in excess strain on the doctor-patient relationship if access to what is perceived as necessary or desirable by healthcare providers is limited by health insurance coverage.

If You or Your Doctor Want
a Second Pathology Opinion

Just as the choice of pathology laboratory could be limited by your health insurance coverage, your choice of pathologist could also be limited by your physician. The pathologist and laboratory that provide the study and the report on your particular case are usually chosen by your gastroenterologist and surgeon or hospital. Rarely are you asked if you would like to choose your own pathologist or laboratory.

Pathology laboratories have been known to make mistakes, so talk it over with your physician if you want to double-check results. It is not uncommon for patients with carcinoma involving a polyp to want another opinion, especially if the biopsy shows that cancer has not broken into the colon wall, but there were cancer cells in the stalk of the polyp. Ask your gastroenterologist to help you arrange for your slides to be reviewed by different pathologists to obtain second and often third opinions on what to do next.

Your tissue samples are kept on glass slides and in paraffin blocks in the laboratory's pathology department. They are part of your medical records, and you can have them sent to another pathologist. Hospital laboratories keep these tissue samples for many years. You will probably have to give the laboratory 24 hour's notice in writing or sign a hospital form so they can release the slides and a written report.

Always be sure to find out ahead of time just what complications you are likely to run into. You will want to know that you are getting the best possible treatment—indeed, the proper treatment.

43

4

CHOOSING PHYSICIANS AND TREATMENT CENTERS

In finding out what to do when you get colon cancer, you will meet many physicians along the way who specialize in various disciplines necessary to your treatment. You will no doubt like some of them and dislike others. You might already have a gastroenterologist who discovered cancer during an endoscopic procedure. If you have confidence in this physician, you might feel confident about specialists he or she recommends. However, before you go ahead and meet these new people, ask your doctor some questions. Ask about the experience, reputation, and personality of the new physician. Sometimes you can be warned in advance that, for example, a particular surgeon seems cold and patronizing, but has a top notch reputation among his or her peers. You will be better prepared to interview this doctor because you will not be expecting warmth and compassion.

FINDING A PHYSICIAN

If you have no primary physician or gastroenterologist, call a health network referral service or medical center in your area, and ask for a gastroenterologist and surgeon with *experience in treating colorectal disease*. There are also books in the reference section of libraries where you can find *board certified* medical specialists. A gastroenterologist will do most of the screening, or it can be done in the gastroenterological endoscopy center of a major hospital.

When you call a doctor for the first time, you have every right to ask for his or her credentials if you cannot find them on your own. Except for physicians over age 60, nearly everyone today is board certified in some discipline of medicine. You will want to be sure all of your treatment team members—surgeon, radiation oncologist, medical oncologist—are board certified. Check the doctor's background by calling the county medical society or by consulting the medical directory at the reference desk of your public library.

First Meetings

Before you go to a first meeting with a new doctor, ask if you can begin your interview with your clothes on before the doctor visits you in the examination room. This way, you get a chance to know the doctor and to ask some questions when you are not naked or partially disrobed and naturally feeling more vulnerable. You want to feel you are meeting on an equal footing, rather than talking with a fully clothed authority figure. When you are dressed, it is easier to question the doctor further or to disagree with something. Unclothed, you might hesitate to object to or press an issue.

When you meet a doctor for the first time, take your medical records and family history with you. Bring a notebook so you can write down questions as you think of them and keep track of information you gather. It is perfectly okay to bring a tape recorder, too, if it helps you remember the answers given and allows you to compare opinions intelligently. This is a cram course with a whole new language and set of information to absorb quickly. If a physician finds a tape recorder distracting, discuss it with him first.

What to Expect

If you feel rushed when you visit a physician for a checkup or procedure, ask for another appointment, so that you have additional time to ask questions and talk. After you get home and think about everything the doctors have told you, it is quite common to think of more questions. Write them down as they occur. There are many things to talk about: your laboratory results, your health history, the side effects of your treatment, your follow-up care. There are big "ifs" lurking in your mind, and you have a right to expect your doctor to help you cope with them. What you want most when you are faced with a serious illness and treatment is help. You want someone to show you the path to cure, to give you only the best information and advice. Some patients do not want to know everything about their disease and its treatment. However, more and more people are becoming informed about health care and believe it is important to be well informed.

If your cancer is advanced, it is even more critical to develop a good rapport with your physician. There used to be a belief among physicians that telling a seriously ill patient as little as possible, and not confronting them with their own mortality, was the most humane way to go. Perhaps that was easier for the doctor, but certainly not for the patient. Today doctors believe that if your cancer is advanced, you have a right to know what to expect, what is the worst that can happen. You should receive comfort and honesty from a physician. Your questions about how long you can expect to live or if you will get well again should be answered in the most simple and direct way possible.

Become familiar with terms such as *cure, remission, five-year survival, recurrence,* and *response.* If the chance of your cancer recurring is 65 percent, for example, you should expect your doctor to explain what that means. Does it mean that in five years, this percentage will diminish if your cancer has not recurred? Nobody can answer that question, and that is what you should expect your physician to tell you. As explained in Chapter 3, the percentages attached to stages are just that. You could be among the 65 percent who get a recurrence in five years or among the 35 percent who are cured forever. Or you could get a recurrence 10 years later. This cannot be predicted. It is wiser to go along one step at a time. Your immediate future can and should be charted.

SURGEONS SPECIALIZING IN COLORECTAL TREATMENT

In Chapters 10, 11, and 12, the chapters about chemotherapy and radiation treatment, you will find information provided to help you select oncologists. And in Chapter 2, with regard to proper screening guidelines, you can find an outline of the qualities to seek out in a gastroenterologist. The surgeon is mentioned here because he or she is usually the first physician to treat you after the gastroenterologist, and your choice of surgeon is directly related to your choice of treatment center where you will spend much time.

Colorectal surgery is complex and requires a great deal of follow-up care. It also has considerable impact on your life, from the time needed for recovery to possibly adapting to the use of colostomy appliances. There are general surgeons as well as surgeons who specialize in diseases of the colon. You are most likely to find these specialists—colorectal surgeons experienced with colon cancer—in comprehensive cancer centers, large medical centers, big cities, and teaching hospitals.

The skill of the surgeon is an extremely important factor in the outcome of colorectal surgery. Complication rates vary considerably, so always find a surgeon who specializes in colorectal surgery and who has been doing so for many years, preferably in a major teaching hospital, where there is access to the latest technology and equipment if complications do arise. The operative mortality for colon cancer surgery is approximately 5 percent, but it can be as high as 17 percent when the operation is an emergency, such as for perforated colon.

Ten Questions to Ask Your Colorectal Surgeon

- What is the goal of surgery?
- Would you describe the operation to me?
- Will I be in pain after surgery?
- What will you do if you find cancer in other organs?
- Will I have a colostomy?
- How long will it take to be fully active again?

- Will I need a special diet after surgery?
- What kind of follow-up care will you provide?
- Will treatment affect my sexuality?
- What are my chances of recurrence?

YOUR TREATMENT TEAM

Several physicians will be involved in your treatment: gastroenterologist, surgeon, and perhaps a medical oncologist. If you have rectal cancer, then possibly a radiation oncologist will be involved as well. And the pathologist plays a critical role behind the scenes. These physicians all lend their expertise and opinions along the way. This is your treatment team, along with an assortment of technicians, nurses, and other healthcare professionals. Keep in mind that you, too, are part of this team.

When you interview physicians on your team, let them know you want the truth, not reassurance, no matter how comforting that might seem. Taking charge of your cancer treatment is the only way you can feel confident that you are doing all the right things to treat it. Do not lose track of the *goal of treatment,* which is to treat your colon cancer and recover.

**Ten Questions to Ask Members of
Your Treatment Team before You Begin**

- What is the stage of my cancer?
- What treatment do you suggest for me?
- Why do you suggest this particular treatment?
- What is the treatment likely to cost?
- What are the benefits of this treatment?
- What side effects can I expect?
- What can be done about side effects?
- What kind of follow-up care is required?
- How will this treatment affect my lifestyle?
- Is this the best medical treatment possible, or are guidelines for treatment set by my insurance carrier?

COMPREHENSIVE CANCER TREATMENT CENTERS

Many medical centers have multidisciplinary treatment teams for specific diseases. Find out if there is a colon (or colorectal) cancer treatment team—often called a cancer conference—at the facility you are considering. This means you could find a gastroenterologist, surgeon, medical oncologist, and other care providers who work together in patient care.

At many university hospitals, a tumor board meets regularly to discuss a multidisciplined approach to cancer patients. The tumor board might include clinical oncologists, radiation oncologists, oncology nurses, and hospital social workers who share information. Your case is very likely to be discussed during such meetings, and this is one way of enhancing the quality of your care. There is input from academic physicians as well as from the clinical physicians and other staff involved in the patient's care. However, this in no way resembles care by committee. Your own physicians are still in charge of your care.

In large cities where you have more choices, you might be able to choose from several well-known teaching hospitals. One good rule of thumb if you must choose between two hospitals is to inquire about their residency training program. Ask if it is approved in colorectal surgery, medical oncology, and radiation oncology. An approved residency training program means there are an adequate number of properly trained faculty members to supervise treatment.

A comprehensive cancer center—usually, but not always, part of a university hospital medical center—will be able to offer you a multidisciplined approach to care usually under one roof. Some of the services available include:

A chemotherapy treatment center
Pathology laboratory services
Pharmacy dedicated to cancer patients
Psychiatric oncology
Cancer hotline for latest information

Nutritional service for treatment and prevention of cancer
Social work program to help you and your family cope with
fears and anxieties
Radiation oncology center
Diagnostic imaging center approved by American College of
Radiology
Diagnostic endoscopy suite
Bone marrow program

TREATMENT CENTER
SUPPORT SERVICES

Many hospitals have clinical nurse specialists who work exclusively with cancer patients and enterostomal (ET) nurses for colostomy patients. They are very helpful during the week or more that you will be recovering from surgery in the hospital. Such nurses teach you how to care for yourself when you get home, and they can recommend support groups and anything else you need.

Written materials and videos are often available. Hospital social workers assist with finding support groups or programs to help families make the adjustments they need. Whenever you need help with anything connected with your hospital stay, seek out the patient services representative. This person can answer questions about the hospital's charges for your care or about any procedures or people involved in your care. The patient services department's purpose is to act as the liaison between you and the hospital, and it is their job to help you.

Patient's Rights

You also have rights as a patient. The American Hospital Association (AHA) published a patient's bill of rights in 1973. All accredited hospitals must accede to this bill, which covers all patient concerns from quality of care, to securing information, to recognizing your right to privacy.

In addition to the right to quality care regardless of ethnic origin, religion, age, or source of payment, the bill of rights outlines what you have a right to expect. For example, you have the right to know the name of any physician involved in your care—as well as other staff members—information about your planned course of treatment, the probable length of hospital stay, and the prognosis for the future. You have the right to participate in decisions that affect your care. You also have the right to consult other physicians.

The right to decline treatment or leave the hospital against medical advice is also yours. If you want to go to another hospital, you have the right to expect the hospital to make that transfer possible. No one outside the treatment team and hospital has a right to see your medical records unless you say so.

The patient services department of most hospitals can provide you with a copy of the AHA patient's bill of rights. In addition, most states have laws concerning rights of medical patients. You can find out about state laws from your patient services department or your state department of health.

Advance Directives

Written or oral instructions about what to do about your treatment if you become unable to make decisions yourself is called an *advance directive*. Hospitals are mandated by law in many states to inform adult patients of their right to make such directives when they enter the hospital.

The advance directive allows you to plan in advance for any eventuality that could leave you unable to communicate with your treatment team. By planning in advance, you can appoint a proxy—a trusted friend or family member—to carry out your wishes if you cannot make them known. Without such advance directives, your family might not be allowed to make decisions for you or to follow your wishes.

You have the right to accept or refuse medical treatment, including life-sustaining treatment. So you can request or consent to treatment, refuse treatment before it has started, or have it stopped once it has begun.

It is always better to have decisions of this magnitude in writing. Your wishes about your treatment and your life can be outlined in what is now known as a *living will*. Whomever you appoint as an agent for your care, to carry out your wishes, can be named in a proxy form that most hospitals will provide.

SHOULD YOU CONSIDER TREATMENT IN A CLINICAL TRIAL?

Before starting treatment, you might want to consider joining a *clinical trial,* a study that uses new cutting-edge treatment to care for patients with your kind of cancer. There might be a clinical trial in progress at the treatment center you choose, or one of your physicians might be involved in such a trial. Many doctors do participate in these trials, so talk with your treatment team. Becoming part of the trial means that your progress through the treatment is monitored closely and that the data are evaluated and included with data from many other patients. Each clinical trial tries to answer certain questions in order to find new and better ways to help cancer patients. If, after the designated number of years, a trial shows that a certain standard works better than others, then it might become the new standard treatment. For example, the chemotherapy regimen combining flourouracil and levamisole for the treatment of colon cancer became standard practice in 1989 after years of study in a clinical trial.

Clinical trials offer the promise of better results than standard chemotherapy. The best candidates for such trials are patients who have advanced cancer, who are not afraid to try new things, and who are fairly young.

Many clinical trials (treatment studies) offer some part of care free of charge. But some insurers will not cover certain costs when a new treatment is under study, so do not consider the trial as a cost-saving measure. Be sure you know what is in your medical insurance policy. Check it to see if there's a specific exclusion for "experimental treatment." Although the medications might be free, you need to find out if your insurance will cover you for side effects. Experimental protocols are not always covered. Many insurance companies handle new treatments on a case-by-case basis, rather than having a blanket policy. You always can ask about their coverage of specific therapies.

Ask your doctor about the experience of other patients in the trial. Have their insurers paid for their care? Have there been any consistent problems? Talk to your doctor about the paperwork he or she submits to your insurer.

For information on current clinical trials for colon cancer, call the Cancer Information Service Hotline at 1-800-4-CANCER. (There is more detailed information about clinical trials in Chapter 11.)

WHAT WILL YOUR TREATMENT COST?

Almost no one asks what treatment will cost. Most patients simply hand over their health insurance card because that is what the hospital or doctor's office asks for. The billing representative does not tell you up front that your week in the hospital will probably cost you more than a year at a five-star hotel on the French Riviera where the food is a heck of a lot better.

Always ask what your treatment will cost. You might, in fact, be responsible for calling your insurance company to inform them about your care. Some insurance companies require you to do this within 24 hours of getting the treatment or it will not be covered. Today's health care system is very complex and is undergoing great change, daily. There are so many health insurance plans that it is difficult to be sure what is covered and what is not.

Patients often have a sense of unreality dealing with large figures, hundreds of thousands of dollars; but make sure you understand what you are paying for and how much it costs. If you are responsible for partial payment according to your insurance coverage, even 20 percent can be substantial.

In addition to the hospital room charges and surgeon's fee, you will be billed for use of the operating room, anesthesia, recovery room, medications, and an assortment of miscellaneous charges. The hospital will give you a list of standard charges for any procedure. You might be asked to sign a consent form, agreeing to pay any charges not covered by insurance. Ask what these charges are so you are not surprised later.

IF YOU ARE IN A HEALTH MAINTENANCE ORGANIZATION (HMO)

Most Americans are now enrolled in HMOs, including Medicare. These are prepaid healthcare plans that combine the functions of the insurance company with those of the doctor/hospital by providing health care for a prepaid annual premium. Most doctors have HMO contracts as part of a medical practice group or as private practitioners who treat HMO members. Doctors are also forming their own HMOs.

Many of these HMOs are improving and offering more choices. Such plans also encourage preventive health care because it is covered in the flat rate. But be aware: The primary care doctor is the one who has the power to decide when you need to see a specialist and which specialist that can be. This is limiting to you because you might not be able to choose a doctor whom you believe will be able to give you the best treatment you need. If you do consult and use a specialist on your own or one who is outside the HMO roster, you might have to pay for it yourself. A limited choice of hospital is also a disadvantage. Finding doctors who will accept a particular HMO, even Medicare, is often difficult.

Some HMO plans are known to be inferior and restrictive. Others are more liberal about paying for some of the cost of physicians outside the plan. Learn what your plan covers. Do not accept treatment you believe is inferior because you are limited by your HMO. Call your insurance company, your physicians, your hospital patient services department. Everything is negotiable if you persist.

If your income is low enough to qualify you for Medicaid, then, in theory, you should have all costs covered. However, this coverage varies from state to state, and some private or community hospitals refuse to accept Medicaid, so patients are sent to municipal or county facilities—not always the best source of care. Medicare might cover you if you are old enough. To check on your eligibility for Medicaid or Medicare, call your local Department of Social Services. If you are over 65, call the Agency for the Aging in your area. (There is more information on health insurance limitations in Appendix 3.)

5

BEFORE YOU BEGIN TREATMENT

Colon cancer treatment is fairly straightforward and offers fewer options than treatments for breast or prostate cancer. Nevertheless, you have to make some decisions now. Generally, if your cancer is invasive and has broken through the colon wall, a section of the colon must be removed. This means major surgery. The second biopsy after surgery will help decide if chemotherapy is necessary.

Both treatment and prognosis of colon and rectal cancer depend upon the depth of invasion of the cancer, the involvement of adjacent lymph nodes, and the presence or absence of distant metastases. Your treatment might involve local excision, polypectomy (a minor surgical procedure to remove the polyp), or open abdominal surgery to remove all or part of your colon. It might also include chemotherapy and, if you have rectal cancer, radiation as well.

GETTING A SECOND OPINION

Suppose you are told that you need open abdominal colorectal surgery. It is quite likely that your gastroenterologist will recommend the best treatment and surgeon if you need one. But do not be rushed. This procedure requires a disruption of your lifestyle, at least a week's recovery in the hospital, and several more weeks of recuperation at home. Now is the time to get all the information and support you need, as well as a second or third opinion.

There are many differences in each individual circumstance and sometimes second opinions are not necessary. Sometimes they are required for your own peace of mind and sometimes they are required by your insurance carrier.

It is very important that you feel you are really getting a second opinion and not just a carbon copy of the first opinion. This can happen if, for example, the first surgeon with whom you talk sends you to another colleague in the same practice, the same hospital or medical center, or even in the same office—just because your insurance requires it or because you desire a second opinion. This is not really a second opinion at all. This is merely fulfilling the insurance requirements so that surgery will be paid for by the insurance carrier. Such second opinions are often shallow and do not really give you any more information or insight into your treatment.

When you ask about a second or even a third opinion, your physician should gracefully encourage you to do this and might even help you know how to seek out other specialists. After all, you are going to sign an "informed consent" agreement before you have surgery. And this means that all the risks, side effects, and procedures have been explained by your surgeon and that you understand!

Keep an open mind when talking with other physicians who review your workup and evaluation, confirm the diagnosis, and discuss available treatment with you. Each time you speak to someone, you will know more, and it might take several conferences to get a good understanding of your situation. This is how you become an informed patient. You know what kind of cancer you have, you know what is in your pathology report, and you might know the stage of your colon cancer. When you talk with doctors, you will have a better sense of what treatment involves. You are extremely vulnerable now, so try to remain objective. As mentioned in Chapter 4, bring someone along for moral support and write down information as you hear it. Write down your questions, too, before you meet with the doctors.

Always bring your medical records with you. It is the most efficient way of communicating important medical information between physicians. The easiest way to handle this is to simply ask for a copy of the report at the time of the procedure. That way you have it available to show other doctors on your team. Physicians are sometimes slow to send copies of reports to others doctors.

By the way, the medical reports from all procedures and biopsies you have had are yours. They are part of your medical records, and you are entitled to have copies. Very often, hospitals are possessive about records and like to make patients think they are not entitled to such records. But the most efficient way to discuss your case is to have your records in your hands at the time of your meeting.

BECOMING AN INFORMED PATIENT—LEARNING THE LANGUAGE

As you have been learning about your disease and your treatment, you have been learning a new language. Now, before you go ahead with treatment, maybe it is a good idea to review some of the basic terminology. The cancerous tumor inside the polyp is usually called a *carcinoma* or *adenocarcinoma*. Some rare and unusual tumors have other names, like *sarcoma*. The *primary* is the origin site of the cancer. If there are other polyps or lesions found at the same time, they are *synchronous*.

For the purposes of diagnosis, your colon, which is about 5 feet long, is divided into right and left sides. Your rectum is an extension of the colon. The spread of cancer from the colon to other areas of the body is called *metastasis*. This can happen three ways: through the lymphatic system (lymph nodes and vessels), through the vascular system (blood), or through direct extension from the primary tumor. For example, the cancer could break through the colon wall and invade the bladder or liver.

Tumor size is measured in centimeters. A 1-centimeter lesion has a one-third-inch diameter and is about the size of a small pearl; two and a half centimeters is one inch; and 4 centimeters is an inch and a half, or the size of a ping pong ball.

Your treatment will be planned in two ways—local treatment and systemic treatment. *Local treatment* focuses on the actual cancer in your colon and can include surgery (polypectomy, colectomy, colostomy, local excision) and radiation. *Systemic treatment* focuses on the rest of your body and is planned if you have a cancer that *can* or *has* spread to other organs. This is chemotherapy with *cytotoxic drugs*—drugs that kill cells.

Many variables guide your treatment planning—size, type, depth of invasion, and location of tumor; cell behavior; lymph node involvement; presence or absence of metastases. Some of these variables will become obvious after initial screening, others not until after surgery, such as whether cancer has invaded your lymph nodes. *Staging* is the sum of these variables and a determination of any evidence that the colon cancer has spread elsewhere. Your treatment will depend on the dynamics of your colon cancer, as well as your age and general health.

When diagnosed with colon cancer, many people panic—and some doctors often rush you into treatment, making everything sound like an emergency. But unless your colon is perforated, you *do* have time to get more information, to talk to others who have been treated, to consider your options, and to make the best choices you can. That cancer has been in your colon for some time, and it can wait a few more days until you make up your mind about what to do.

Colon cancer is treatable, and in many cases potentially curable. Treatment is improving all the time, and survival rates increase every year, so take the time to find the best treatment available. Trust your instincts. You will know what is right for you if you learn all you can about what is available.

Be sure you understand the purpose of all treatment procedures. For example, treatment is usually aimed at curing the disease (curative) or at slowing its growth and reducing pain (palliative). Understand, also, how each procedure will effect your lifestyle in the near and distant future.

IF YOU HAVE OTHER MEDICAL CONDITIONS

The majority of colon cancer patients have reached an age at which they often have other medical conditions to cope with. These conditions can be affected by colon cancer treatment, so it is a good idea to think about this before you begin. If you have a preexisting heart, lung, or neurological condition, your health care must be communicated among physicians, to avoid duplication and waste.

You will need to know how much of your care will be transferred to your oncologist if you are getting chemotherapy. If you are getting a numbness or tingling in your left side, who do you call? Your oncologist? Your primary care physician? Your cardiologist? Is it from the chemotherapy, or is it from your heart condition? One of the pitfalls of having so many physicians is never being quite sure whom you should call with a question about a problem.

Patients tend to call whichever doctor answers the phone. It is a good idea to find doctors who are not only competent, but who will respond to your needs quickly. If you cannot reach your oncologist but you can reach your gastroenterologist, for example, then ask that physician to put you in the hands of someone who can help with your immediate problem.

It is a good idea to always remind your colon cancer treatment team members about your other doctors. Also, copies of reports will be needed by all of them during treatment and follow-up care. It is your responsibility to follow up on reports. Call your surgeon and ask, Did you get a copy of the report from my oncologist?

Physicians fax reports to each other all the time, but the speed with which they do this can vary with the physician and the physician's staff. Some doctors will make sure a report is forwarded the day it is requested. Others might not be as prompt. The easiest and least stressful method is for you to get copies of your reports from your doctors as they are generated and carry them around with you.

As soon as a procedure is done or a report completed by your physician, get a copy. When you have multiple conditions, always ask for copies of your records so you have the information to show whichever doctor needs to see it. This is the most efficient way.

FINDING THE EMOTIONAL
SUPPORT YOU NEED

Most people know very little about colon cancer, and it can be devastating news not only to you but to your family and friends.

They might think the worst—that they will lose you. Many patients try to protect their families from the details, but this makes everyone's anxiety worse. Talk openly and honestly with your family and friends. Now that there is more awareness and activism about cancer, there is a growing network of information and support—for you and your family. In fact, your family should get involved and begin their own screening procedures, because their own risk of colon cancer is probably greater.

The cooperation of your family is essential to your recovery. If your activities must be restricted, for instance, tell them how this will affect your participation in family life and what you would like them to do for you. How will it affect them? Just as successful treatment is from a medical team, the same team effort will be needed in your recovery with your family.

Explain to family members what is going on. If they hear it from others, they might be misinformed. People close to you might feel helpless when they cannot do anything to help or fix the situation. Plan ahead and assign friends or members of your family to various jobs, such as getting the information from the doctor after surgery, checking the messages on your answering machine at home, picking up things you might need in the hospital, bringing food, and so on.

This is also a good time to look for a support group to prepare yourself emotionally and to talk with others who have been through the same experience. Your hospital social worker might be able to give you information.

If you know you will be having a colostomy, talk with your doctor and nurses about special education and training. You can contact the United Ostomy Association and arrange for someone who has a colostomy to come and talk with you. (Very often the hospital will do this for you.) There are Colostomy Clubs all over the country, and they provide their members with practical and emotional support. (There is more about such support in Chapter 16.)

Many cancer centers now have specialists in psychiatric oncology, a program designed to help cancer patients cope with their disease and their treatment. Some medical centers also offer a variety of programs to help patients reduce the stress and pain involved in their treatment. These include biofeedback, relaxation techniques, and even hypnosis. There is much available, so take advantage of everything.

A CHECKLIST OF THINGS TO DO BEFORE BEGINNING TREATMENT

Colon cancer treatment affects your work, family, and lifestyle. If you have open abdominal surgery, for example, you might be in the hospital for a week, and it will take several more weeks before you are recovered enough to go back to work or resume a normal lifestyle. Unless your surgery is an emergency, you should have a reasonable amount of time to rearrange your work and social schedule and to get ready for the surgery and your recuperation.

Presurgery Checklist

- Ask and get answers to such practical questions as: Will you be able to wear your own clothes? Will you be able to see a newspaper each day? Should you bring some books or your portable CD player? Should you bring your own toiletries and medications needed for other conditions?
- Designate a friend or family member to talk with the surgeon immediately after your surgery and to contact your other physicians about the results.
- Find out what support systems are available to you.
- Arrange your work schedule so you will know how much time off you can count on, and when and how you are likely to return to work. Arrange for someone to handle details of your work that might be necessary in your absence.
- Plan for someone to care for things at home while you are in the hospital.

If you have taken care of all these matters before you go in for surgery, you will not have to worry when you need to stay focused on letting yourself get well.

With all the changes in the health care system in recent years, doctors have not quite figured out whether the system is becoming more complex or less complex. They hope that after all the confusion, what will evolve is the best possible delivery of health care to everyone who needs it, the best treatment for the patient. But right now, the system is in confusion, so you need to be especially alert to what you are dealing with.

It is important to understand, too, that the healthcare system neither begins nor ends with doctors. Patient education is a necessary part of the growing responsibility for you, the patient, to assume some of the care and decision making for your treatment.

Your doctors, too, are learning new ways to practice medicine and to communicate with patients. Now that doctors have a dialog with patients, you, too, are required to participate. Ask questions and tell your doctor if something is not clear. Together, you can provide the best possible treatment.

If you have read and understood everything in this book so far, you should feel more confident now as you enter the next phase, treatment and recovery.

PART II

TREATMENT

6

SURGICAL TREATMENT: LOCAL EXCISION, POLYPECTOMY

Before the development of fiberoptic endoscopic tools in the 1970s, plain abdominal X rays, barium enema X rays, and rigid sigmoidoscopies were the only diagnostic procedures doctors had to find out if there was an obstruction in the colon. And although the obstruction showed up on the X-ray film, there was no way of knowing if that obstruction was benign or malignant. When a patient went to sleep in the operating room, he or she knew only that there was something in the colon. It could be a benign polyp or a stage D carcinoma. The patient could wake up to hear devastating news or get a big smile from the surgeon.

Polyps in the early stages of colon cancer were rarely removed in the past because the polyp usually grew to large or dangerous proportions and metastasized before it was discovered. Today, through fiberoptic endoscopic screening and biopsy, a patient knows before entering the operating room that cancer is present; so, on awakening after surgery, the patient needs only to hear if the cancer appears to have spread to other organs or if it has been totally removed by surgery.

AN OVERVIEW OF SURGICAL TREATMENT

Both treatment and prognosis of colon and rectal cancer depend upon the depth of invasion of the cancer, the involvement of adja-

65

cent lymph nodes, and the presence or absence of distant metastases. In general, surgical treatment cuts away the tumor, then follows with a course of adjuvant chemotherapy to catch any possible lingering cancer cells or to prevent their return. In cases of rectal cancer, radiation is often added after surgery to rid the area of the threat of metastasis.

There are slight variations on these treatments that will be explained as the chapter goes along. But it is most important to be sure you fully understand the rationale behind the treatment your physicians recommend. Within certain boundaries, colon cancer treatment should be individualized after taking into account a patient's extent of disease, lifestyle, and needs, not to mention age, occupation, and personal philosophy. For example, a police officer who wears a gun in a holster would do well to avoid a colostomy if possible because the holster would press against the colostomy appliance. However, if it cannot be avoided, a surgeon can measure that officer in uniform and while going through the motions of drawing a gun, reaching for handcuffs, and so on. Often, the surgery can be planned so as to avoid any undue stress on the appliance.

Surgical treatment—local excision and polypectomy or colon resection—is usually recommended for all Stage A, B, and C prognoses, unless the patient is at an extremely high risk for surgery; that is, the patient has other medical conditions, such as heart disease, drug addiction, or obesity that could add to the risk of anesthesia or the trauma of open surgery.

Following surgery, chemotherapy with fluorouracil combined with levamisole or leucovorin will be offered to virtually all patients with Duke's Stage C cancer and sometimes for Duke's Stage B cancer, but this is an area of controversy. Some physicians believe surgery is sufficient for these stages because the chance of the cancer having spread elsewhere is so low that putting the patient through the expense and possible discomfort of chemotherapy treatment is not practical. (For more on chemotherapy treatment, see Chapter 6.)

Colorectal surgeons usually do not recommend surgery for Duke's Stage D cancer unless resection is required to control bleeding, relieve pain, protect adjacent organs, or prevent bowel obstruction. At this advanced stage, surgery might also be required to remove parts of other organs, such as the liver or ovaries, where the cancer might have spread. Chemotherapy or radiation treatments in patients with *inoperable* Duke's Stage D cancer have been marginally effective. But radiation therapy might be useful in relieving pain when the colon cancer has spread to the bones. Clinical trials of chemotherapy or biological therapy are also an option for patients at this stage.

Although it is not a general practice, some physicians try to shift the Duke's Stage by using preoperative radiation, sometimes in conjunction with chemotherapy, to shrink the tumor and thus to improve surgical results with a lesser stage cancer. This is sometimes successful. It is not common to give preoperative radiation to change a classification, but it has been done, so it is mentioned here. The radiation treatment carries with it other potential problems. If your doctor suggests preoperative radiotherapy, ask many questions about the goal of treatment and get at least one more opinion.

Radiation treatment is primarily used for rectal cancer that can present more complications because of its location. The rectum is surrounded by fat and by a network of nerves and blood vessels at the base of the spine that control sexual and voiding functions, among a host of others. If cancer is low in the rectum, a local excision can be done through the anus. Otherwise, rectal cancer requires an abdominal-pereneal resection with the creation of a colostomy. This might be done with or without preoperative chemotherapy and/or radiation. (See Chapter 5 for information about radiation treatment for rectal cancer.)

Treatment for Early Colon Cancer

Most early colon cancers—Duke's Stage A and B—can be cured by simply removing the cancer. This is done during a colonoscopy, for a colon cancer in a polyp, or with surgery. As mentioned earlier, if a polyp is found during a sigmoidoscopy, it is important to wait until the patient can come back for a colonoscopy to determine if there are any other polyps in the colon. If cancer is present in a polyp of the colon or rectum, the extent of its involvement must be evaluated, but some general guidelines exist about what to do next.

- If the cancer only involves the tip or mucosa of the polyp, the cancer, in essence, has been cured by the polypectomy and no further surgery is indicated. This situation is known as carcinoma in situ. Surveillance colonoscopy should be performed in 6 to 12 months.
- If, in the opinion of the pathologist, the cancer is moderately or well differentiated, if it extends below the mucosa of the polyp but does not involve the blood vessels or lymphatics of the polyp stalk, the cancer has probably been cured by removal of the polyp. Open abdominal surgery with resection of the involved section of the colon is *not* indicated because the surgical risk is generally regarded as being higher than the risk of finding any residual cancer in the colon. Follow-up surveillance colonoscopy would be scheduled at 6 to 12 months after the removal of the polyp.
- If cancer is found to involve the resected margin of the stalk of the polyp, then cancer remains in the colon wall despite removal of the polyp, and surgical resection of the involved area of the colon is appropriate if the patient can undergo surgery. Repeat colonoscopy is performed 3 to 6 months later.
- If the cancer has involved the blood vessels or lymphatics of the polyp, there is a risk that residual cancer cells might be present in or might have spread to the wall of the colon. Many physicians would recommend a segmental surgical resection of the colon if the patient is a good operative risk. If residual cancer is found in the colon wall at the time of surgical resection, repeat colonoscopy for surveillance might be done in 3 to 6 months. If no residual cancer is found in the surgically resected colon wall, colonoscopy would be done in 6 to 12 months.

WHEN POLYPECTOMY
IS ALL YOU NEED

If cancer has not reached the edges of the polyp, it is not likely to threaten other organs. Research has shown that, even when cancer is in the tip of the polyp, the likelihood that it has spread elsewhere is so minimal that polypectomy is generally sufficient for cure.

However—and this is a big *however*—some physicians still prefer to remove the section of colon that contained the polyp because they are uneasy about the possibility that there could be a micrometastasis in the colon wall or stalk of the polyp that would be discovered years later. Many patients, too, would rather have it out and be sure, even though colon resection means open abdominal surgery requiring an extended hospital stay and weeks of recuperation.

If you and your doctor decide that a polypectomy is sufficient, even with the presence of invasive cancer cells, then you both need to assume some of the responsibility for possible undertreatment with this decision. You must also take into consideration your own ability to maintain surveillance. Are you sure you will be diligent about getting the necessary and frequent colonoscopies and fecal occult blood tests, and possibly other tests, to monitor your colon for possible return of cancer? Consider these questions seriously.

Each case is unique. An 80-year-old patient with other health problems might be at greater risk from open surgery and anesthesia than from a possible colon cancer metastasis—in that case, polypectomy is preferred treatment. But a 55-year-old in the prime of life could easily withstand surgery. This is a tough call and is one of the areas of controversy in colon cancer treatment, so it is important for you to discuss it carefully with your doctors. Your biopsy report, your age, and your lifestyle are all factored into your treatment plan. If your gastroenterologist and pathologist believe you do not need surgery, be very sure you feel comfortable with that prescription. If not, this is a good time to get another opinion from another gastroenterologist, pathologist, or surgeon. Take your pathology report and slides with you.

In general, a polypectomy is sufficient treatment for a cancerous polyp with invasive cells if:

- The polyp was not excised in piecemeal fashion.
- Blood vessels and lymphatics do not appear to be involved.
- The colon wall is not invaded.
- Cancer cells are not poorly differentiated.
- No cancer shows at the margins of the resection (site of the removed polyp).

If cancer cells have invaded the polyp stalk or the lining of the colon wall or if there is evidence of blood vessel and lymphatics involvement, a colectomy (colon resection) would be a wise choice of treatment.

The Polypectomy Procedure

Preparations for polypectomy are the same as preparations for colonoscopy, so you can refer back to Chapter 2 and read the section on screening for diagnosis. Be sure you have a complete understanding of the procedure, so ask as many questions of your physicians as you need.

Before asking you to consent to the procedure, your doctor will caution you and tell you what to do about the risk of possible bleeding following the procedure. Bleeding can occur during the procedure, but the doctor can easily control this. Hemorrhage following polypectomy often requires hospitalization and might even require a blood transfusion.

Expert polypectomy technique must be applied by the gastro-enterologist, and the site will be recorded and might be marked with sterilized india ink so the surgeon can find it if you should need open abdominal surgery. A careful written assessment and description of the polyp and its location must also be supplied by the gastroenterologist. Because the colon is so flexible, the surgeon might not always find the polyp exactly where it shows up in the pictures taken by the endoscopic camera.

The polyp is encircled with a wire snare and then an electrocau-terizing current passes through the endoscopic tube, and the polyp is removed. This might be all the treatment you need. However, it is critical to follow through with a biopsy and monitored surveillance with periodic colonoscopy to survey the entire colon for additional polyps. If you had one polyp, you are at higher risk to develop more.

After a thorough biopsy of the polyp is made by the patholo-gist, the information is communicated to your other physicians. Your gastroenterologist, pathologist, and surgeon all must cooper-ate to assess the information about your colon cancer. Even with great care, it is possible for some polyps, especially sessile polyps without stalks and those removed piecemeal, to be inaccurately assessed for margin of resection and depth of invasion.

After a Polypectomy

After the uncomplicated discovery and removal of an adenomatous polyp of the colon or rectum, you will need to follow up with a colonoscopy usually at two- to three-year intervals. And in the years when colonoscopy is not performed, your physicians might recommend that you have a complete blood count to watch for any change in tumor marker levels and that you are tested for hidden blood in the stool. If the polyp was particularly large or if multiple polyps were present, your physician might modify this and recommend more frequent screening with colonoscopy.

The goal of this surveillance is to detect and remove polyps that recur at the same site or form at different sites in the colon and rectum—some practitioners have likened this to "weeding the garden." Then your doctor might want a follow up colonoscopy in another month or within three months. Another biopsy of the site of the removed polyp might also be prescribed. If no more cancer is found, then an annual colonoscopy is usually all you need.

The need for such surveillance cannot be overemphasized, because once you have had a cancerous polyp, you are at three to four times greater risk of developing a second primary cancer of the colon. If another polyp develops and shows cancer, it can be removed the same way, or a surgical colon resection can be done. If cancer is detected early, even the second time around, it can usually be cured with surgery.

LOCAL EXCISION FOR RECTAL CANCER

Because there is so much fatty tissue between the rectum and the nearby organs, including the network of sacral nerves that control sexual function and bladder control, it is often assumed that microscopic tumor cells could be lurking in this congested area, ready to invade other parts of the body. Although sophisticated colorectal surgery can now spare the sphincter muscles and sometimes, the vital sacral nerves as well, the general surgical rule is to cut away as wide a margin as possible—just to be safe.

If you have a small rectal carcinoma of less than three centimeters in diameter (1.25 inches), if your biopsy reveals that the cells are well differentiated (not fast growing), and if the lesion is mobile when it is examined, you might have the option of a local excision without open abdominal surgery and lymphadenectomy.

This surgery can be performed transanally or with a posterior proctotomy. In many of these cases, deep resection and/or fulguration (burning away the tumor in multiple, staged attacks, with electrical cauterization) of the base of the polyp can be performed under general or spinal anesthesia, through the anus, with the surgeon using a variety of instruments designed to shave the tumor and its roots.

Local excision is often substituted for open abdominal surgical resection of the involved section of colon. Many factors will help decide if this approach is appropriate for you. A second opinion would also be appropriate for this situation.

Radiation therapy is almost always a follow-up to this surgery to eliminate any possible lingering cancer cells in the pelvic area. When radiation is expected to follow rectal surgery, the surgeon will mark the area to be irradiated with large metal clips. This provides a guide for the radiation therapist in locating the tumor bed. (See Chapter 10 for more about radiation treatment.)

7

SURGICAL TREATMENT: PARTIAL AND TOTAL COLECTOMY, COLOSTOMY

The surgical principles of colon cancer treatment have been known for more than a century, and despite enormous improvements in detection, surgical technique, antibiotics, anesthesia, and colon preparation, the basic curative treatment has not changed much: Cut away the diseased portion of the colon, and reconnect the two healthy sections. This is called surgical resection, resectional surgery, colectomy, or hemicolectomy. Surgical techniques for rectal cancer are different, and they will be discussed later in this chapter.

It is currently possible—but seldom practical for cure—to resect the colon without fully opening the abdomen by using laparoscopic techniques. This technique involves inserting a tube through the abdominal wall, and with the aid of cameras and video screens performing surgery inside the abdomen by manipulating tools at the end of the tube. However, this laporoscopic surgery is not yet widespread in curing colon cancer. For one thing, the surgeon cannot see and feel the adjoining abdominal organs, especially the liver, and this is an important step in evaluating the disease and its treatment. In addition, the technique for this surgery requires formidable skills that few surgeons and medical centers currently have. So far, laparoscopic surgery has been primarily used to perform palliative therapy to reduce pain in patients with advanced colon cancer. But there are important clinical trials in progress.

ABOUT OPEN ABDOMINAL SURGERY

Traditional colorectal surgery is open abdominal surgery under general anesthesia. It includes not only resecting the colon, but removing lymph nodes for analysis and investigating nearby organs, such as the liver, for signs of cancer. The length of colon removed depends on the size of the cancer and its location. Your surgeon will want to leave a wide margin on either side of the tumor, usually four centimeters (1.5 inches). Where the two healthy parts of the colon are sewn back together is called *anastomosis*.

Removing the entire colon would be a *colectomy*, and removing the colon and the rectum would be a *proctocolectomy* resulting in an *ileostomy*. There are many labels for colon surgery, although they are all the same surgery. These include *transverse colectomy, sigmoid colectomy,* a *subtotal colectomy,* and *ileoproctostomy.* This last might be prescribed if your cancer is potentially curable but adenomas are scattered in the colon and if you have a family history of colorectal cancer in first-degree relatives. None of these definitions are important to you because doctors call them by other names as well. What you do need to know is what your surgeon plans to remove and what will be left behind.

If your tumor is in the sigmoid colon (the descending colon), you will be treated with a left hemicolectomy, the most common type of colon cancer surgery. If your cancer is in the cecum, a larger section of colon is often removed on the right because there is only one blood vessel attached to that portion of the colon. If that vessel is severed, the colon itself could die without proper blood supply.

Sleeve resection is the simplest resection. It is done in cases of a very small tumor, or with a frail person who will not tolerate open surgery well. The cancerous section is cut away, the healthy sections rejoined, and that is all. No lymph nodes are removed, nor are other organs investigated.

GETTING READY FOR SURGERY

Within the two weeks before surgery, you might be scheduled for preoperative tests such as a chest X ray, an EKG (electrocardiogram), and blood tests to check your general health and to be sure you are able to tolerate surgery and general anesthesia. You will want to interview the anesthesiologist, and you will be asked to sign consent forms.

- **Chest X ray.** This is always required before surgery to be certain that you have no pulmonary obstruction or signs of metastasis in your lungs.
- **EKG (electrocardiogram).** This is a normal part of the routine before surgery to check your heart function and to detect any abnormalities that might affect you during anesthesia and surgery.
- **Blood tests.** A complete blood count (CBC) checks for iron deficiency anemia and the need to correct this before surgery. Another very important blood test is the carcinogenic embryonic antigen (CEA) assay to measure your carcinoembryonic antigen level before removing the primary tumor. This test is a tumor marker and becomes important after surgery as a way to watch for any signs of recurrence. If CEA levels are elevated, it is a warning for physicians to look for possible metastasis of the colon cancer. The level shown before surgery will be used as a baseline from which to gauge any changes that might occur after surgery.
- **A CAT scan.** A CAT scan of the abdomen to search for metastatic disease is not routinely done before colon cancer surgery because your surgeon will be able to examine your liver and other organs during the operation. However, if you have rectal cancer, a CAT scan of the pelvis is valuable in locating possible intrapelvic metastasis and also aids in planning radiation therapy before or after surgery.
- **Interview with the anesthesiologist.** The risks of general anesthesia have decreased dramatically in recent years as drugs and techniques have improved. However, ask the anesthesiologist which drugs will be used, and be forthcoming about *any* drugs

you are taking. For example, aspirin affects platelet function and can be associated with increased bruising.

- **Consent forms.** You will be asked to sign consent forms for anesthesia, for biopsy, and for many procedures you encounter along the way. But do not sign anything until you know exactly what will happen. This is what *informed consent* means. Ask what kind of anesthesia they plan to use, how it will affect you, and any aftereffects you can expect. Write the answers down. Also ask the anesthesiologist if he or she has any particular concerns about your surgery. Ask your surgeon about the potential side effects of surgery and about possible removal of other organs.

IF YOU HAVE CURRENT MEDICAL CONDITIONS

As mentioned earlier, other medical conditions should be brought to the attention of all of your physicians before colon cancer treatment. Some medical conditions present risk factors for surgery.

A recent heart attack could mean no general anesthesia could be given within three months of that attack. Obesity and cigarette smoking could also preclude general anesthesia. Your health will have impact on your follow-up treatment, too. A diabetic receiving chemotherapy could have a low-blood-sugar reaction if he or she is unable to maintain proper diet. If a patient is using insulin, its dosage might need to be adjusted. A patient with a heart condition would not be able to tolerate certain of the cytotoxic drugs used in chemotherapy.

Some risk factors for surgery include:

- Stress
- Smoking
- Obesity
- Excess alcohol consumption
- Use of recreational drugs
- Use of steroids
- Poor nutrition
- Chronic illness of the heart, lungs, liver, or gastrointestinal tract
- A recent illness

These conditions might increase your risk of surgical complications. Ask your colon cancer treatment team members to consult with your family doctor or other medical specialists who treat you so they will know how treatment for colon cancer might affect conditions for which they are treating you.

TALKING WITH YOUR SURGEON

Ask your surgeon if he or she will see you before you go into the operating room. You might want some reassurance, so ask about the operating-room routine. How long you can expect to be in there? Where you will go when the surgery is finished? How many people will be working on you? Will you feel any pain?

Be sure you know in advance which family member or friend will be able to talk with your surgeon immediately after your operation so the family can know how you are and let your other doctors and family members know. Should that person meet the surgeon in the recovery room? in the waiting room? Will your surgeon tell that person honestly what he or she found while examining your abdominal cavity? Some surgeons might hesitate to say they saw cancerous lesions on other organs until they have done a biopsy, but they should tell your relative that they are checking on any lesions they might have discovered. This is important for the peace of mind of your family and will avoid frustration later when you wake up in your room and have no information.

If you have not already done so, it would be wise to ask your surgeon what he or she will do if cancer *is* found in other organs. You might want to be prepared to live without your ovaries, for example, and know about it in advance. Make sure you understand all the implications before you consent to surgery.

Also find out how long your family is likely to be waiting around during your surgery. Sometimes a surgery is delayed for some reason that has nothing to do with the patient, and nobody from the operating room staff comes out to tell the family. As they sit in the waiting room for hours, they worry and wonder what is taking so long. They will fear the worst.

DESIGNING YOUR SURGERY TO FIT YOUR WORK AND LIFESTYLE

One of the most important things to discuss with your surgeon is how your surgery—especially location of incisions—can be adapted to your lifestyle. As mentioned earlier, a police officer was able to have a colostomy designed to allow him to continue at his occupation and wear all of the equipment involved in the job. The surgeon measured this patient as he went through all of the motions involved in his work and while wearing all of his equipment, especially the gun holster belt that crossed his abdomen. The location of the colostomy, and colostomy bag, was shifted to accommodate his work.

The importance of letting your surgeon know about your work and lifestyle cannot be overemphasized. Unless your surgery is an emergency, there is ample time to discuss and possibly plan ways to accommodate you. Many occupations involve activity or equipment that could affect colostomy: a bus or cab driver, for instance, who must wear a seat belt for long periods of time, a telephone line person or window washer who wears a safety harness, an airline pilot, an athlete whose physical positions could have an effect.

TALKING WITH THE SUPPORT MEDICAL STAFF

The hospital might routinely assign special cancer care nurses to you after surgery, or they might assign an enterostomal (ET) nurse if you have a temporary or permanent colostomy to help you adapt for functioning on your own at home. But find out in advance what to expect. Will the floor nurse come when you need him or her, or should you hire a private nurse for the first day or two? This is particularly important if you have other health conditions to cope with or if you are very frail or elderly. Before you are admitted, go to the nurses' station on the floor where you will stay and ask the nurses how they feel about it—or ask a friend or family member to do this.

The amount of time floor nurses can give you depends on the size of the hospital, the number of nurses available in your unit, and how highly skilled they are in dealing with equipment and procedures required in your postop care. If they feel extra care is needed, they can give you a roster of private duty nurses available, both registered nurses and licensed practical nurses. Consider whether you will want three nurses, each working an eight-hour shift right after your surgery, or if you would like one nurse for the same time each day, say from 8 A.M. to 4 P.M., to help you get up and walk around, to administer medications, and to change dressings.

MAKING SURE YOUR DOCTORS ARE COMMUNICATING

The majority of colon cancer patients are of an age where other medical conditions might be affected by colon cancer treatment. If you have ongoing medical problems, it is a good idea to be followed before, during and after your surgery by your primary care doctor, internist, or other subspecialist, treating, for example, your heart disease, hypertension, or diabetes. These doctors should enjoy a good working relationship with your surgeon.

Let your family doctor—or doctors other than your surgeon—know when surgery is planned. They might want to visit you in the hospital after surgery to see how you are doing from their perspective. Depending upon your medical conditions, these physicians would naturally be concerned about how your surgery has affected your other medical conditions. They might want to monitor your blood pressure, heart, kidney function, respiratory tract to watch out for pneumonia, and reactions to the medications they have prescribed for you, as well as any reactions to medications given during and after your surgery. For example, a gynecologist would want to know if ovaries were removed. A urologist would be concerned about any rectal surgery that created problems of incontinence or impotence.

Before you have your surgery, you should meet and talk with any specialists you will be seeing later, such as your medical oncologist or radiation oncologist or possibly a gynecologist or urologist if you will be facing incontinence or sexual dysfunction from surgery. If the extent of your disease is unknown before surgery, you might not want to incur the cost of these consultations unless you know you will need them. However, you might feel it is better to confront all of this before you progress into treatment so that you understand how your treatment and recovery will affect your lifestyle. Once you know that you can treat and deal with these complications and that your lifestyle can eventually return to normal, or near-normal, you will not feel hopeless and depressed about what the future holds. Going through treatment in a negative frame of mind can affect your treatment and recovery.

SHUTTING DOWN THE DIGESTIVE SYSTEM

To assure successful surgery, it is important that your intestines be empty and clean. This is called "mechanical bowel prep" for elective surgery, as opposed to emergency surgery, and begins two days before surgery. In the past, a patient would come into the hospital the night before for this preparation, but now you do it at home and come in the morning of your surgery all ready to go to the operating room.

Your doctor will give you detailed instructions, but the procedure is something like this: Two days before surgery, you will stop eating solid food and begin a diet of clear liquids only. You might be required to drink citrate of magnesia or the lavage used for colonoscopy to clear out any remaining waste material. This substance turns fecal matter to liquid and flushes it from your body. You might also be asked to give yourself a self-administered enema the morning of surgery to remove any residual fecal matter. (Refer to Chapter 2 for the preparation for colonoscopy.)

The night before surgery, you might be required to take antibiotics, such as arythromycin or neomycin, to kill bacteria remaining in the colon. Another dose of intravenous antibiotics might be given to you immediately before and right after surgery.

IN THE OPERATING ROOM

Although this is a high-anxiety period, you probably will not be given any sedatives or tranquilizers to relax you before surgery. The anesthesiologist is better able to control the depth of anesthesia necessary for the surgery with less risk if other drugs are not in the way.

Operating rooms are necessarily chilly in order to keep the multigowned surgeons and staff cool during the lengthy time in an enclosed area with high-powered lights and other equipment. But you will be covered with a warm blanket after you are prepared. It is important that you be kept warm to fight off infection. A drop in body temperature inhibits defenses against germs, decreases the blood flow to the skin, and lowers the supply of oxygen necessary to fight infection. Cold also interferes with blood clotting. Because anesthesia will interfere with your body's ability to regulate its own temperature, it is important that you be kept warm.

THE SURGERY

The nurses and anesthesiologist get you ready, paint your abdomen with antiseptic, and cover up the rest of your body with sterile drapes. Pneumatic boots will be put on your legs to help maintain good circulation while you are asleep and to minimize the chance of developing a blood clot in your legs. A Foley catheter will be inserted to drain off any urine that collects in your bladder. During this time, the anesthesia will begin to make you relax, and your surgeon might come in and talk with you so that you are feeling reassured as you drift off to sleep. Colon resection surgery and lymphadenectomy take about two hours. Formation of a colostomy might take slightly longer.

Surgical Incisions

Incisions are generally drawn down the center of your abdomen, often from just above the navel to the pubis. Sometimes they begin higher up, closer to the sternum if the cancer is high in the colon. A transverse incision on the right or left side of your abdomen is sometimes used for right- or left-sided lesions. The layers of muscle, fat, and skin of your abdomen are separated and clamped to expose the organs inside.

Because the colon stretches and is free-floating, the cancer is not always found exactly where it showed up on the colonoscopy, so the surgeon must explore. What the colonoscopy shows is merely a guide. Gross examination—what the surgeon can see and feel—is very important in this kind of surgery. Once the incision is made, clamps are placed above and below the diseased portion of the colon and the cancerous portion of the colon is cut out.

Variations on the surgery depend upon your particular case and your surgeon.

Exploring the Abdomen

The peritoneum is the membrane covering the abdominal organs and abdominal wall. This membrane is also cut through during surgery. Infection of this membrane is called *peritonitis,* so any leaking contents of the colon must be vacuumed away. The wide incision gives the surgeon a critically important view inside your abdomen (peritoneal cavity) and the chance to feel (palpate) your liver and inspect it for signs of metastases. (If a metastasis was suspected, a CAT scan of the liver might already have been done.) The most critical areas of concern are the other parts of the intestines, the liver, and the pelvis. All should be examined, as should the full length of the large bowel. This should be palpated along every inch. In women, the ovaries will also be examined. All adjoining organs can be explored so the surgeon will know that if extensive disease is found, the nature of the surgery might change—it might call for a less radical resection than would be provided for a cure, and chemotherapy might be needed later.

Lymphadenectomy

Lymphadenectomy is the surgical removal of lymph nodes, which are crucial indicators as to whether the cancer cells have spread and if you will need chemotherapy after surgery. When the colon section is removed, the surgeon will also cut out a wedge of the mesentery. This is a film of tissue that contains blood vessels and lymph nodes that drain the colon. It is attached to the back of the abdomen wall and supports the intestines. Because the lymph nodes drain the colon, that is where cancer cells would go. Not only is lymphadenectomy critical for staging, it is also therapeutic. If any lymph nodes do contain cancer, their removal has eliminated additional cancer from your body.

Most surgeons now remove all the lymph nodes that drain the resected piece of colon. There is no prescribed number of lymph nodes to look at, but at least 10 should be removed if possible. The number can also depend upon the location of the resection. For instance, there tend to be more lymph nodes near the cecum—the right side of the colon—and fewer near the sigmoid colon on the left.

Each removed lymph node is examined carefully by the pathologist. However, even if the lymph nodes are negative—containing no cancer—a small number of patients with invasive colon cancer can develop metastatic disease. Once the surgeon removes the fatty tissue containing the lymph nodes, the pathologist presses through the tissue to free all of the lymph nodes for inspection.

Colon resections *without* lymphadenectomy are called for only when the patient is known to have widespread metastasis or is too frail, making further surgery risky.

Removal of Other Organs

If curing your colon cancer is the goal of surgery, then your surgeon might remove any nearby organs that show cancer. This might also be done as a preventative measure. For instance, from 2 to 8 percent of women with colon cancer will eventually show metastasis to the ovaries. For this reason, the ovaries are sometimes removed as a preventive measure. Such prophylactic oophorectomy is considered routinely for post- or perimenopausal patients, but it is not clear that this is necessary for premenopausal patients because the incidence of colon cancer in this age group is rare.

If cancer has invaded nearby organs, this is not necessarily a dismal prognosis. As mentioned earlier, isolated lesions can be safely resected from the liver. Be sure to talk with your surgeon about this possibility in advance. He or she cannot remove any organ without your permission, and you will probably have been asked to sign a consent form before surgery.

Margins of Resection

Studies of colon cancers indicate that submucosal tumors rarely spread more than 2 centimeters (about 1.3 inches) beyond the visible disease. Most surgeons try to cut out enough colon so that 4 centimeters (about 1.5 inches) of healthy colon remain on either side of the tumor. About a foot of colon is removed. Some suggest leaving as much as 2 inches of clean margin to avoid local recurrence.

The size of the section removed is also determined by location of the blood vessels. There are several that supply blood to the colon, but there are more blood vessels on the left side—the sigmoid area—and there is only one on the right—the cecum area. That means a much larger piece of colon will be removed from the right side in order to maintain blood supply. If too short a piece of colon is removed and the blood vessel is cut, the adjacent colon might die. Proper resection of the colon requires preservation of adequate blood supply via the mesenteric blood vessels to the remaining colon. To accomplish this, the surgeon is bound by certain surgical techniques that ensure this. Surgical care must be individualized to each patient.

Reconnecting the Colon

Because your colon stretches like a rubber band, it can be shortened and reconnected without too much impact on your digestive system. If anything, a shortened colon reduces constipation. Your colon will eventually adapt to the new shorter length.

The inner and outer layers of your colon are stitched or stapled together. Surgeons have their own preferences for the method used. The standard method is stitching the inner layer with a watertight seal of catgut, which eventually dissolves, and the outer layer with silk thread, which is permanent. Layers of your abdominal muscle, fat, and skin might be sewn together with stitches or staples. These details depend upon the location of your resection and your surgeon's preference.

After colon resection surgery, you will spend some time in the recovery room until your doctor is certain that you have tolerated the surgery and anesthesia and that there appear to be no complications or excessive bleeding. When you wake up, you might find tubes up your nose or bandages down your front. You might feel abdominal soreness, and you might be very thirsty. How to cope with all this? Read Chapter 9.

8

SURGICAL TREATMENT: RECTAL AND RECURRING CANCER

About 20 to 25 percent of cancers of the large intestine are rectal cancers, and these are most common in people between the ages of 50 and 70. Many patients with rectal cancer delay coming in for treatment because they think they have hemorrhoids. And sometimes they do—but that does not mean they do not also have a carcinoma. *Hemorrhoids* are varicose veins that protrude from the anal lining and are aggravated by constipation and straining to pass stool.

One 70-year-old man, who delayed visiting a gastroenterologist until he noticed large amounts of blood in his stool, insisted to the doctor that his hemorrhoids were bleeding. A sigmoidoscopy and biopsy revealed that he had a large cancerous tumor in his rectum. When surgery and adjuvant chemotherapy was prescribed, the man insisted that he just wanted the hemorrhoids removed.

This patient delayed treatment every step of the way because of his insistence that he did not have cancer and that he would not be able to "wear the bag," meaning the appliance needed with a colostomy. After many months of procrastination, and after losing weight and showing many other signs of cancer, he finally consented to surgery but still resisted the recommended follow-up chemotherapy.

TYPES OF SURGERY

There are a variety of techniques that allow removal of the tumor while preserving the sphincter muscles, thus avoiding colostomy. The rectum is about 5 inches long and surrounded by fat, which is a particularly fertile breeding ground for cancer cells. Any invasion greater than Duke's Stage A requires a wide excision, usually combined with abdominal resection and colostomy. This is not usually required for similar cancers higher up in the colon.

Anterior Resection

Cancer of the upper rectum is easier to control and is usually treated with an anterior resection. This can be appropriate if the growth is more than two and a half inches from the anus. This procedure removes the tumor and some cancer-free bowel on either side. Then the remaining rectum is joined to the colon with a surgical stapling system. A staple gun is inserted into the rectum through the anus, where it delivers a ring of tiny metal staples that hold the edges of the rectum and the colon firmly together.

In general, a rectal tumor can be treated with an anterior resection, without a colostomy, if the lower edge is more than 8 centimeters (about 3 inches) from the anal verge in a woman or more than 9 to 10 centimeters (4 inches) from the anal verge in a man. When cancer is in the lower part of the rectum, the entire rectum and the anus must be removed, and a colostomy done.

There are also a host of potential complications because of the location of the rectum. Nerves needed for sexual potency and continence are generally destroyed during surgical treatment for rectal cancer. To compound this, blood vessels that men need for penile erection are often destroyed in radiation treatment that commonly follows rectal surgery. Sometimes the coccyx at the base of the spine is removed in order to expose the rectum and facilitate resectioning.

A patient with a small rectal cancer tumor, even in the distal 6 centimeters, might refuse a proctectomy and colostomy because of the possible complications and changes in lifestyle that come with this operation. Or the patient might not be a suitable operative candidate. In this case, a local transanal excision of the tumor might be considered. This might be a less than optimal treatment, leaving the patient with a risk of recurrence.

Colostomy

This procedure is performed when removal of the tumor requires removal of the rectum. A colostomy is a new opening through which waste matter can pass. Only about 15 percent of colon cancer patients, or one in seven rectal cancer patients, receive a colostomy.

When the colon and rectum is removed, the small intestine—the ileum—is passed through an opening—a stoma—in the abdomen wall, and the result is a total colectomy or total proctocolectomy, which results in an ileostomy. The new opening in the abdomen wall becomes the stoma. Waste is eliminated through this stoma into a sleeve that can be emptied directly into the toilet or into a pouch fastened to your body. Vast improvements have been made in colostomy appliances, and it is not as difficult to live with as it was when the bags were bulky and made of rubber, which did not conceal odors very well.

Sometimes, a temporary colostomy is needed in order to give the lower colon and rectum time to heal after surgery. A second operation is performed later, and the healthy sections of the colon are joined and the stoma removed. Then bowel function returns to normal. (For more information, see Chapter 16, Living with a Colostomy.)

SIDE EFFECTS OF RECTAL SURGERY

Radical colorectal surgery to the rectum, usually has side effects that cause lasting changes in your lifestyle. All of these side effects must be explained to you by your surgeon before you consent to the operation. The most serious side effects result when some of the sacral nerves are cut away. These nerves, centered at the base of the spine, innervate the thighs, buttocks, and muscles and skin of the legs and feet, as well as of the anal and genital area. They cannot be restored after surgery, so this is one reason why it is so important to understand exactly what your surgery means.

When the nerves are severed, it can cause sexual dysfunction in men. Less common, but also possible in men, it can cause urinary retention; that is, the nerves that make possible the reflex that allows the release of urine do not work.

Radiation treatment for this area of the body can also produce problems. Radiation is almost certain to destroy the blood vessels necessary for penile erection. Chemotherapy can limit the ability to function of the muscles in the genital area.

Sexual function can be restored in a variety of ways. Be sure you know all you can about these side effects so that you can understand how you can treat these problems after your surgery. (Chapter 18 deals with reversing the sexual side effects of colon cancer treatment.)

SURGICAL OPTIONS FOR METASTATIC AND RECURRING COLON CANCER

When colon cancer is advanced, the more common treatment would be chemotherapy to help reduce pain and improve the quality of life for the patient. Surgical resection of the colon would not cure the cancer, but it might be considered necessary to prevent further obstruction of the colon, to repair damage such as perforation, or to stop bleeding.

However, if colon cancer has spread to the liver, there are surgical options for further treatment. If a single hepatic metastasis or group of lesions in a single lobe of the liver is discovered and there is no other evidence of metastasis, then surgical resection of the liver is considered the best option and might provide a long-term, disease-free, clinical course. Left untreated, a lesion of the liver would soon be fatal.

Colon cancer usually spreads first to the lymph nodes and then to the liver through the blood vessels. The liver is the most common site of metastasis. It is also the first site of distant spread in about one-third of patients with recurrences and is involved in more than two-thirds of fatalities. Colon cancer rarely spreads to lungs or lymph nodes around the clavicle or to less common areas, such as bone or the brain, without first involving the liver. The most notable exception to this generalization is in patients with a primary tumor in the lower part of the rectum. Tumor cells from lesions in that area can spread through the blood vessels around the spine and vertebra and travel up to the lungs and supraclavicular lymph nodes at the juncture of neck and shoulders.

Resection of the liver has been performed in appropriate patients for more than 30 years, and 5-year survival rates are about 25 to 35 percent. This surgery is considered appropriate for patients whose primary tumor is controlled or controllable, who have fewer than five metastases in the liver, and who show no other sign of colon cancer. In experienced hands, the operative mortality for this operation is less than 5 percent. However, only about 5 percent of patients who had colon surgery are suitable for this procedure, and they are generally younger, otherwise healthy patients. Elderly people or those with heart disease or other chronic conditions, might not be good candidates. Talk with your doctor or chemotherapist to learn what your options are.

More and more, patients with isolated metastatic cancer of the liver can be identified early by the monitoring of their carcinoembryonic antigen tumor marker levels—CEA assay—through blood tests. Tumors do recur in about one-third of these patients.

If your cancer has come back in only one part of the body, treatment might consist of an operation to remove the cancer. If the cancer has spread to several parts of the body, your doctor might prescribe either chemotherapy or radiation therapy. You might also choose to participate in a clinical trial testing new chemotherapy drugs or immunotherapy. (See Chapter 4 for information on clinical trials using new chemotherapy drugs.)

PROPHYLACTIC SURGERY FOR FAMILIAL ADENOMATOUS POLYPOSIS

About 1 percent of colon cancer patients have inherited the disease, usually at a very young age, from a genetic condition known as familial polyposis syndrome (FAP). This syndrome causes thousands of polyps to develop along the entire inside of the colon. Because there is no known way to prevent familial polyposis from developing, the only treatment is to remove the colon so polyps cannot develop. This prophylactic surgery is performed in adults as soon as the disease is diagnosed and in children when they reach their late teens. It is unnecessary to operate sooner because most people with this syndrome do not develop the cancer until they are 20. The treatment in young people is almost always accomplished easily without complications by using either the standard method or the J-pouch method.

The Standard Method

This procedure requires removal of the entire colon and the joining of the small intestine directly to the rectum. Once the patient's digestive system has had a few months to adjust to the shortened intestine, normal bowel function resumes.

The J-Pouch Method

This method was first used in the 1980s and is still a highly specialized procedure. The surgeon removes both the colon and the mucous membrane of the rectum, without harming the rectal sphincter muscle. This muscle will be joined to the lower end of the small intestine, which will be transformed into a sac-like reservoir or pouch to imitate the reservoir function of the rectum.

Surgeons seem to like the J-pouch for FAP and chronic ulcerative colitis (CUC) patients, but it is less used in a colon cancer resectioning. For this, it is necessary to operate twice. During the first surgery, the colon is removed and a J-pouch created, even though it cannot be used right away. The small intestine is brought outside onto the surface of the abdomen—an ileostomy—and for three months, stools will be eliminated through this stoma into a bag. Then, the ileostomy will be removed, and the feces allowed to pass through the anus again.

In rare cases, where the patient has already developed cancer of the rectum before the detection of polyposis, the only possible treatment is colostomy. About two months after this operation, all polyps in the rectum are removed by polypectomy during a sigmoidoscopy, which will be required from one to four times a year for the rest of the patient's life to immediately remove the new polyps that will continue to appear. Otherwise, the patient is at risk for the development of rectal cancer.

The J-pouch method eliminates the risk of developing new polyps in the rectum, but it takes the patient 6 to 12 months to attain normal bowel movements. Once a year, the pouch will be examined with an endoscope.

When FAP is found and treated early, the patient lives a perfectly normal life with no urinary or sexual system disorders. Women who have had a J-pouch or standard surgery for familial polyposis have just as much chance of getting pregnant and going through childbirth without complications as any other woman, although a Caesarean birth is advisable after a J-pouch operation. In addition, all examinations, except for the X-ray study of the colon, can be carried out safely. (Chapter 19 provides more about protecting your family from colon cancer.)

9

RECOVERING FROM SURGERY

After colon cancer, you will usually be in the hospital for five to seven days, although you will not need to stay in bed the entire time. In fact, your surgeon might want you up and walking by the next day—or even that night if your surgery took place early in the morning. Compression boots might be kept on your legs for another day or so to keep circulation normal. A Foley catheter will continue to drain urine from your bladder.

You will be fed intravenously the first two days until your digestive system recovers from the anesthesia and begins to function again. You will feel thirsty but probably not really hungry. Although your digestive system is not yet working, there are still gases and fluids circulating in that system without a purpose now, and you might have a nasogastric tube through your nose and into your esophagus to drain these fluids.

Recovering from colon cancer surgery is like recovering from any major surgery. Follow your doctor's instructions, take it easy, watch out for infection, and resume your normal routine as soon as possible. The following are some of the conditions with which you might have to cope.

CONTROLLING PAIN

Pain will be moderate to severe for the first 24 hours and gradually ease off. You might also feel pain from your incision as it heals, but in general, after about four days most of the pain should be gone.

Gas pain occurs because of lack of coordination of your intestines after surgery. It is important to acknowledge your pain—don't grin and bear it. Suppressing pain can cause shallow breathing, and this can cause some of the air sacs in your lungs to collapse.

The good news is you will have some control over your pain relief. In modern medical centers, patients now manage their own pain with the PCA (patient controlled analgesia) system. Medications such as morphine and dilauded are expressed from a nearby machine whenever you press a button. If you need more pain relief, you can press the button and get some more. The PCA system is regulated to release a certain amount of pain medication per hour so there is no fear of overdosing.

You might find it painful to sit up or to cough or sneeze for a few days. Anything that calls on your abdominal muscles, which are understandably stressed, could make you feel sore. Several layers of your colon and your abdomen—muscle, fat, skin—around your incision must knit back together.

CARING FOR YOUR INCISIONS

For the first few days, great care will be taken around the wound site to avoid contamination and infection. Your surgeon will want to examine the wound site to check it, so bandages will be changed at least once a day. Once the wound has begun to heal, usually after one or two days, they might leave the dressing off to allow the circulation of air to help in the healing. A hard ridge will form along the incision as it heals, and the ridge will gradually recede after several months.

Once you get home, you can bathe or shower normally, but wash around your wound gently with mild, unscented soap. Call your doctor if you notice any redness, swelling, or oozing. Sometimes a warm heating pad can relieve pain around the incision.

If you had a colostomy, you will have a stoma, which needs special care. (There is information on stoma care in Chapter 16, Living with a Colostomy.) Your surgeon will probably want to see you a week or two after surgery for suture removal and to check on the healing process.

ACTIVITY AND EXERCISE

You might feel wobbly the day after surgery, so ask one of the nurses or one of your visitors to help you walk short distances—down the corridor, for instance, or to the hospital lounge. Walking helps get your body functioning, and it is also a good cure for gas pain.

After open abdominal surgery, take special care not to put pressure on your abdominal muscles until your incision is well healed. However, regular activity and walking is good for your entire well-being. There might be limitations on lifting anything that will call on your abdominal muscles. Ask your surgeon for detailed instructions. If he or she says no heavy lifting, ask what is considered heavy. Obviously, you will not do situps or pushups, but you might bend down to pick up your newspaper from your doorstep and pull your abdominal muscles. Ask about the best technique for getting up from a bed or chair and how to bend and lift and reach and stretch—standing on your toes and reaching overhead, for example, could pull your abdominal muscles.

RESTORING YOUR DIGESTIVE SYSTEM

Nasogastric Tube

Most colon cancer patients do not need the nasogastric (NG) tube. This tube is used to drain fluid from your stomach until your digestive system kicks in again and takes over. The tube is connected to a canister on the wall near your bed where the suctioned fluid is collected and monitored. Because bile and acid are still released into your intestines, even though they have nothing to work on, they must be suctioned away from your digestive system. This is like removing sludge from an engine. Removing this fluid helps to prevent you from having nausea until bowel function resumes.

Because the NG tube is passed through your nose, through your esophagus, and into your stomach, it can be uncomfortable.

94

The tube can make you gag, or it can hurt your chest. For instance, if you cough, you might feel it rub against the back of your throat. Be sure to ask for a nurse or physician to adjust the tube if it is not comfortable.

Foods and Diet

You will be fed intravenously and get only ice chips or a bit of water, if you can tolerate it, until the second day after surgery. Then you should be able to drink clear liquid—meaning liquid you can see through—such as apple juice or broth. A regular diet will probably begin on your fourth day with soft foods like applesauce and Jell-O®, but it will probably be at least seven days before you have solid foods. This gives your colon time to heal without putting excess strain on it. When patients begin to feel better, they think about food, and this can make the liquid and soft diets pretty frustrating. Friends and family members might want to bring you more interesting liquids or soft food from home, such as ice cream shakes, yogurt, or juices that might not be available at the hospital.

Before you leave the hospital, a dietitian will probably meet with you and suggest a low-residue diet for the first few weeks after surgery. With less fiber, your healing colon will not be irritated by too much roughage. Your diet will probably be adjusted according to how it affects you. For instance, you might have diarrhea for a little while after surgery, so add rice or tea to your diet to help bind foods and stabilize loose stool.

Your postoperative diet is likely to be reviewed and modified during your outpatient follow-up visit with your surgeon. Be prepared to ask questions and review in detail how you are doing in terms of diet and bowel function. Often, a high-fiber diet is empirically recommended to help provide for a normalization of bowel function. There will be some period of trial and error in the weeks following surgery until you are back to normal. Here are some general guidelines.

- Try only one food a day that you have not eaten since surgery.
- Avoid foods that cause diarrhea or constipation.
- Take small bites and chew well.

- Drink plenty of water, at least eight glasses a day.

(Chapter 15 deals with diet and its effect on colon cancer.)

Return of Normal Elimination

Urination could be painful the first few times after surgery once the urethral catheter is removed. If a large section of colon was removed, you might have loose stool and possibly have some bleeding at first, but, within two weeks, bowel function should be normal. For a while, you might feel sensitivity in the section of your colon that was operated on as fecal matter passes.

WHAT TO EXPECT AFTER A COLOSTOMY

In the past, the hospital stay after a colostomy was about three weeks, or until doctors were certain the patient could manage at home. Now, the emphasis is on home care and patient responsibility. This means arranging for a home-care nurse who comes daily for at least one week to check your vital signs, to see how your wound is healing, and to continue teaching you how to manage your colostomy appliances and procedures. Gradually, the visits are cut back as the patient and family assume the responsibility.

In most large hospitals, a specially trained enterostomal therapy (ET) nurse will work with you after a colostomy and help you learn how to cope with the special appliances. (You might have received some information in advance of surgery.)

You will need to get used to having a *stoma,* an opening in your abdomen. The stoma is made of membrane, which looks much like the inside of your mouth, and can secrete mucous. It has blood vessels, so it can bleed if it is irritated. No matter how well prepared, the initial sight of the stoma is a shock to most patients, almost like a slap in the face. But with help from the nurse specialists and support groups, you and your family can learn to adapt. Some hospitals arrange for an ostomy representative to visit you in the hospital before as well as following your surgery.

If you had a total colectomy, your feces will now pass directly from your small intestine through the stoma and into the colostomy pouch. Because there is no longer a colon to remove water from waste matter and make it solid, you will have liquid feces.

If any problem becomes severe or causes pain, be sure to report it to your ET nurse and doctor. (Everything you want to know about diet, buying appliances, treating infections, bathroom techniques, intimacy, and physical activity can be found in Chapter 16, Living with a Colostomy.)

GETTING READY TO GO HOME

It will take you a couple of months to feel normal again, so before you leave the hospital be sure to get written instructions about taking medication, how to care for your incisions at home, and other follow-up care.

A Checklist of Things to Ask about before You Go Home

- What pain medications to take if you need them.
- Signs of infection to watch for.
- Bathing: When to take showers or tub baths.
- When to have follow-up visits with surgeon and/or gastroen-terologist.
- When to call the doctor if something is bothering you.
- How often to change your dressing.
- Clothing to wear to avoid irritating your incision or stoma.
- When to begin normal physical activity and exercising.
- What to eat and not eat while recovering.
- What to expect from bowel function; how to identify a problem.
- Home healthcare nurses: Will you need them, and what do they provide?
- Colostomy appliances: How to use and care for them.
- When to begin getting chemotherapy or radiation.

10

RADIATION TREATMENT
FOR RECTAL CANCER

L ike surgery, radiation therapy (also known as *irradiation* or *radiotherapy*) is a local treatment—it treats only the area it directly touches. It is rarely used for colon cancer because radiation into the abdomen has not proven successful and can be toxic when combined with chemotherapy. However, radiation therapy plays an important role in the treatment of patients with Duke's Stage B and Stage C rectal tumors, and it is quite effective in curing the cancer or preventing recurrence.

There are several ways of using radiation to treat rectal cancer. It can be used before surgery to shrink the tumor, or it can be used after surgery to kill any lingering cancer cells. Researchers are studying the benefits of using it both before and after surgery—the sandwich technique—and even during surgery.

Some physicians have used radiation before surgery to try to shrink the tumor sufficiently to allow its removal and resection. But, for most patients, the best time for radiation treatment appears to be after surgery. First, surgery is not delayed for the four to five weeks needed to administer radiation. Second, a sphincter-sparing operation, if feasible, is more likely to succeed when the bowel has not been irradiated. And because the stage of disease is not always determined until after surgery, patients with early Duke's Stage A or Stage B or widespread Duke's Stage D disease are spared unnecessary treatment.

Nearly 50 percent of recurrences in rectal cancer occur in the pelvis because the rectum is so close to so many pelvic organs. Surgeons cannot achieve a wide, tumor-free margin during resection for rectal cancer as they can higher up in the colon where they can cut out as much as a foot of colon and stretch two healthy sections back together without harming nearby organs.

When rectal cancer metastasizes, it often shows up in the prostate, the bladder, or the vagina and causes extreme pain. It might also invade the sacral-area nerves that control sex and voiding. The rectum is five inches long and is surrounded by fat and immediately adjacent to a rich supply of lymphatics. This enhances the early spread of cancer cells into surgically inaccessible areas. But radiation *can* get to those areas, and this is one of the reasons for its importance in treating rectal cancer.

Radiation, which has been around for over a hundred years, uses approximately 500 to 1,000 times more energy than what is used with regular X rays. This high dosage from high-energy equipment kills all the cells in its path—good and bad—so they cannot grow and multiply. However, new healthy cells will replace those lost. Radiation can be applied externally, by aiming X-ray beams at the treated area, or it can be done internally by implanting radioactive isotopes.

Radiation therapy is strictly regulated by federal and state nuclear regulatory commissions. The dose of radiation delivered to the rectal area at most institutions is between 4,500 and 5,000 rads (radiation absorbed dose) or cGys (centigrays). A boost dosage of an additional 1,000 to 2,000 rads is often delivered directly to the tumor bed in the last part of the treatment. This varies with the philosophy of the institution.

Small metal clips—like staples—are inserted at the margins of the surgical bed during your surgery. This marks the edges of the area where the tumor was. But they will remain in your body forever. These clips define the tumor bed to help the radiation oncologist decide where to deliver the boost. When a CAT scan is done as part of the treatment planning, these metal clips can be seen on the scan and a final radiation field can be very accurately placed, based on the clips' position. The boost dose uses the same type of radiation. It is just more focused.

THE TREATMENT PROCESS

Most radiation treatment begins four to six weeks after surgery and is given daily from Monday through Friday for five to seven weeks. It is painless—just like getting an X ray—but you might feel some discomfort lying in the particular position you must maintain while the radiation is penetrating. While you lie down on a table in the radiation room, the highly trained and state-licensed technicians set up the machinery to the proper angle, position you accurately according to computer, and administer the dose of radiation.

Radiation Therapy

The radiation is sent into your rectum through your pelvic area for only a few seconds, although you might be in position for five minutes or more. After a week or two, your pelvic area might swell and your skin may become slightly pink to a deep red in the treated area. The intensity varies with each individual and skin type.

The boost is the final phase of radiation treatment—usually given during the last two weeks. A boost directs a dose of radiation directly into the tumor bed. There are two ways to do this: externally, by using the radiation machine, or internally, by implanting radioactive particles into your body. Cost and cosmetic results are similar. Most patients get the external boost.

It is always best to lead as normal a life as possible during the weeks of treatment. However, radiation can make you tired and possibly nauseous, so do not expect to function at your full capacity. Rest when you need it. Most patients do, and, if you can schedule treatment for early mornings or late afternoons, you can work with little interruption to your day.

Follow-up Care

When radiation therapy is completed, expect to have a routine checkup within two months. This will include a physical examination of the rectum to check the aftereffects of treatment and possibly a transrectal sonogram.

You should also see your surgeon at six-month intervals. You might alternate with your medical oncologist if you are taking cytotoxic chemotherapy. This close follow-up procedure continues for five years while the potential for recurrence is highest.

WHEN RADIATION IS COMBINED WITH CHEMOTHERAPY

In treating rectal cancer, radiation therapy might be used in combination with chemotherapy or used before or after chemotherapy. One study showed that compared with the same dose of radiation used alone, this combined regimen of radiation and chemotherapy reduced the recurrence rate by 33 percent and the death rate by 29 percent.

Two new regimens of radiation in combination with the chemotherapy drug flourouracil (5-FU) resulted in a significant reduction in the rates of local recurrence, distant metastasis, cancer related deaths, and all deaths. Apparently, either by continuous intravenous infusion or rapid injection of 5-FU throughout the period of radiation therapy, the local recurrence of rectal cancer was reduced.

There are two adjuvant chemotherapy and radiation therapy regimens reported to be effective in Duke's Stage B2 and Stage C rectal cancer. The first begins 22 to 70 days after surgery. The chemotherapy is administered by rapid injection daily for 5 days, starting over every 28 days. Then, on day 56, or after the second cycle of chemotherapy, radiation is given for 5 days a week for 6 weeks. The two therapies continue to be administered in a combination of days and dosages until treatment is finished.

The second regimen is the same, except that when administered with radiation, the chemotherapy is given by continuous infusion throughout the period of radiation. (See Chapter 11 for information about chemotherapy treatment.)

SIDE EFFECTS OF RADIATION THERAPY

The side effects of rectal radiation therapy have a lasting impact on your lifestyle, so it is important that you understand what they actually involve, and how you can correct these side effects. Because of the location of vital blood vessels at the base of the spine, it is impossible to prevent damage during radiation treatment. Even if the nerves in this area were spared by conservative surgery, the effects of radiation to those blood vessels cannot be prevented.

Chronic damage to the small bowel or bladder is uncommon, but men might become impotent because radiation damages the blood vessels that carry blood to the penis for an erection. Similarly, vessels that carry blood to the genital area in women during sexual arousal might not function as well and result in vaginal dryness.

However, this does not mean that you will no longer have a sex life. It simply means that men will have to adapt to new ways of achieving an erection, and women may need to use a lubricant during intercourse. It is very important to discuss this openly with your physician and your partner so you can learn how to deal with it. (See Chapter 18 for ways to reverse the effects of treatment.)

Radiation therapy to the pelvic area can cause the following side effects:

- **Gastrointestinal symptoms.** Nausea, vomiting, cystitis, and diarrhea. To relieve these problems, you might be able to change your diet or to take medications. Be sure to ask your doctor about this.
- **Hair loss in the pelvic area.** This could be temporary or permanent, depending on the amount of radiation used. In some patients, this does not happen at all.
- **Skin irritation.** Red, tender, dry, and itchy skin in the pelvic area. These symptoms might be alleviated by not wearing clothes that will rub against your skin. Loose-fitting cotton clothes are best. It is important for you to take care of your skin during radiation treatment, but do not use any creams or lotions without checking first with your doctor. Some compounds could actually irritate your skin more. Use clear warm water instead of soap and creams in the treatment areas, patting dry very gently. If the area itches, consult your radiation therapist. Prescription creams or a light sprinkling of cornstarch might help. Avoid heavy lotions. They might leave a coating on your skin that can interfere with your treatment and cause further irritation. Try a light, water-based lotion instead.

- **Fatigue.** You will probably be very tired during the weeks of radiation therapy, but you will be able to work and carry on your normal activities. This is good for you emotionally, as well. However, see if you can shorten your work day or take a rest in the middle of the day.
- **Cancer risk.** The risk of getting cancer again as a result of radiation therapy is negligible. There is no evidence that radiation will increase the risk of cancer. Nor is there any evidence that it increases the risk of any other cancer, such as lymphoma.

(The information in Chapter 12 will help you deal with some of these side effects.)

WHERE TO GO FOR RADIATION THERAPY

Radiation therapy is most often done in comprehensive cancer centers and teaching hospitals and more commonly in large cities or urban areas. Because they treat so many more patients, attract more experienced physicians, and use up-to-date equipment, big-city teaching hospitals and comprehensive cancer centers often provide the best treatment. You will want to know that there is a CAT scanner available and a physicist on staff to handle problems that might arise with the equipment. Your colorectal surgeon will refer you to a radiation oncologist and radiation treatment center. If your surgeon does not feel the need to send you to a radiation oncologist experienced in colorectal cancer, it might be wise to go find one yourself. You might feel better with a second opinion—you can call the American Cancer Society, the National Cancer Institute, or the American College of Radiology. Libraries, cancer hotlines, and support groups are also good sources of information.

Choosing a Radiation Oncologist

A radiologist is a physician who specializes in using radiant energy in the diagnosis and treatment of disease. A radiation oncologist is a radiologist who is specially trained in treating cancer. This physician will probably be recommended by your colorectal surgeon, but here, too, do not accept a radiation oncologist with whom you do not feel comfortable and confident. Ask questions about the physician's background and experience in treating colon and rectal cancer. You want to know about his or her board certification, number of years treating the illness, and how your treatment will be administered.

Will the radiation oncologist personally supervise your treatment or will technicians handle the daily routine? If the latter is the case, expect your radiation oncologist to talk with you and examine you at least once a week during your course of treatment. Be sure to ask about the side effects. Is the goal of treatment to cure your cancer or slow it down? Also ask about the chance of receiving this treatment again in the future, should the cancer metastasize. How often will you be able to talk with this doctor? Can you call with questions?

As a professional group, radiologists tend to be very focused, and some seem to be more interested in the technology than in the human or emotional aspects of their patients. There are many exceptions to this, and it is up to you to draw out the physician. Ask your doctor for some examples of how other patients managed their radiation therapy.

Expect your radiation oncologist to consult with you and other members of your treatment team, to examine you thoroughly before administering your radiotherapy, and to review your medical reports.

Questions to Ask the Radiation Oncologist before Treatment

In order to understand what your treatment involves and how it will affect you, here are some questions to ask:

- What is the goal of this treatment?
- How will the radiation be given and who will give it?
- What kind of side effects can I expect and what can I do about them?
- Can I choose the time of day that I get my treatment?

- How will treatment effect my sexuality?
- Will treatment leave me incontinent?

For more information on radiation treatment for colon or rectal cancer, call the National Cancer Institute for their booklet *Radiation Therapy and You*. Also call them for information on radiation treatment centers.

THE COST
OF RADIATION THERAPY

A complete program of radiation therapy for rectal cancer can cost tens of thousands of dollars in a large medical center in the Northeast. This includes treatment planning and 35 treatments. Most of that is a technical fee, and about one-third is the professional fee. Most medical insurance covers this cost in the treatment of cancer, Medicare covers 80 percent of the cost, and Medicaid covers it all. If you are covered by a health maintenance organization, be sure you understand the rules governing coverage for radiation treatment.

11

WHEN YOU NEED CHEMOTHERAPY

Colon cancer cells are resistant, and they respond only to variations on two drug regimens that have been in use since 1989, when a particular combination of drugs dramatically increased survival rates. The course of chemotherapy for colon cancer most commonly takes a year, but each case is unique. Sometimes six months might be enough, and sometimes it might take longer. The good news is that the side effects are generally not as intense as they can be with drugs used for other cancers. In the very near future, researchers expect the next breakthrough to involve an entirely new class of drugs for chemotherapy treatment of colon cancer.

CHEMOTHERAPY DEFINED

Chemotherapy is the use of any chemical, drug, or steroid in a *systemic* treatment, that is, treatment involving your entire body. The drug goes through the bloodstream and kills cancer cells. It also kills normal cells, and that is why the side effects can be so potent. But the normal cells grow back, and there are ways to cope with side effects.

Every case of colon cancer is unique because there are so many variables and because colon cancer cells are so unpredictable. Colon cancer cells can move around and show up very soon somewhere else in your body, or they can remain dormant until years later. But, in general, if you are at high risk for metastatic colon cancer, with one or more positive lymph nodes or an aggressive (high-grade) cancer, your treatment team might prescribe chemotherapy.

Chemotherapy is standard treatment for Duke's Stage C colon cancer and sometimes—although it is still controversial—for Duke's Stage B cancer. When planning chemotherapy treatment, your medical oncologist will consider many factors, including your age, the size and type of your tumor and its grade (aggressiveness), and the number of lymph nodes involved. Other indicators can include the results of many of the pathology studies of cell behavior.

Adjuvant Chemotherapy

When chemotherapy is used before surgery, it is called *neoadjuvant therapy*. This is sometimes used in treating rectal cancer in order to shrink the tumor before surgery. When chemotherapy is used after surgery to cure cancer or to keep it from spreading, it is called *adjuvant therapy*. The goal of adjuvant chemotherapy is to protect against recurrence in patients with tumors in Dukes' Stages B and C. Although approximately 70 percent of patients who undergo resection surgery appear to be cured, about one-third of this group will eventually develop the disease again. So adjuvant chemotherapy reduces the chances of that happening. Adjuvant therapy is distinct from treating known metastatic disease with chemotherapy. Then, it is called *palliative chemotherapy,* and the goal is to slow the spread of cancer or relieve pain. Be sure to talk with your oncologist about your chemotherapy before you start. It is important to find out what is expected from your treatment. You need to know if the purpose is to cure the cancer, to protect you from recurrence, to shrink the tumor, or to relieve pain.

Reactions to Chemotherapy

Chemotherapy has long been associated with nausea, hair loss, and other difficult side effects, but these vary in intensity for each individual. Some patients experience only mild reactions. Generally with adjuvant chemotherapy, the most powerful side effects of nausea and vomiting last for a few days after each treatment, then subside. Hair loss *(alopecia)* and fatigue might last until the end of the treatment. Treatment might also bring on early menopause, but most women in treatment for colon cancer are postmenopausal. The libido might be diminished in men and women, but this will return after treatment. Men may also experience difficulty with erection because of muscle weakness caused by the medications.

CYTOTOXIC DRUGS USED FOR COLON CANCER

Cytotoxic drugs—drugs toxic to cells—have a variety of mechanisms for action. Some interfere with DNA to inhibit growth. Some act as antibiotics or steroids. Some work to strengthen your own immune system. Fluorouracil, also known as 5-FU, is the most prevalent drug used in colon cancer treatment. It incorporates itself in the cell's normal DNA and, masquerading as a normal building block, prevents the malignant cells from dividing. Cytotoxic drugs can be used alone or in combination and for a variety of time periods. Combinations try to take advantage of the different mechanisms and thereby kill the most cells.

Fluorouracil (5-FU) and Levamisole

Fluorouracil was used by itself in the treatment of colon cancer beginning in the 1970s, but studies showed better survival rates when it was combined with levamisole for Duke's Stage C colon cancer. Adjuvant chemotherapy with this combination of drugs reduced the incidence of recurrence by 41 percent in three large clinical trials. This combination has been in general use since 1989, and it improves the five-year-survival rate from 50 percent to 62 percent and reduces deaths by one-third. Researches still do not know, however, whether this improvement represents an increased cure rate or a delayed rate of recurrence.

Fluorouracil is called a *fraudulent* substance because it fools the cells into absorbing it, and thus blocks certain food vitamins and nutrients needed for cell growth. Levamisole is the first immunity-stimulating agent approved in conjunction with chemotherapy. The combination of 5-FU and levamisole has been associated with the entire gamut of side effects: nausea and vomiting; anorexia as well as weight gain; hair loss; dry skin, rash, and itching; diarrhea; fever and chills; bruising and bleeding; mouth sores; and darkening palms and nails.

With this combination chemotherapy, more than half the patients in one clinical study had nausea and diarrhea, although fewer than half experienced vomiting. About 25 percent of them had hair loss. A very small percentage of patients show neurotoxicity—signs of impaired thinking—but this usually returns to normal after chemotherapy.

The combination of 5-FU and levamisole can elevate the alkaline phosphatase in 40 percent of patients. This is sometimes related to a rising CEA level and with fatty liver, as demonstrated by CAT scan or biopsy. These changes always raise the question of metastatic cancer in the liver, but they are otherwise reversible.

Fluorouracil and Leucovorin

This combination is used generally for six months and most commonly for rectal cancer, although some oncologists use it for colon cancer, too. Leucovorin is folic acid, or Vitamin B-1. It binds to the enzymes and makes the 5-FU more toxic to cells. These drugs attach themselves to the ever-multiplying cancer cells and block their multiplication. This combination has decreased the recurrence rate by 30 to 35 percent.

Various regimens of levamisole and leucovorin are still being studied in clinical trials.

WHO GIVES YOU CHEMOTHERAPY

A medical oncologist is a doctor of internal medicine who specializes in the treatment of cancer using medications as therapy. Oncologists are generally internists, although some are physicians from other disciplines, for instance, a pediatrician might specialize in childhood cancer.

As an internist, this physician is trained to understand internal systems—the cardiovascular, pulmonary, endocrine, digestive, and renal systems—and is able to know how chemotherapy effects those systems. To become an oncologist, an internist needs to complete three more years of medical training called an oncology fellowship. During this period as an oncology fellow, a physician is studying the latest literature on chemotherapy and working with treatment teams on the latest cancer treatment.

Expect your medical oncologist to consult with you and other members of your treatment team, to examine you thoroughly before administering your chemotherapy, and to review your medical reports, especially the pathology report, to find out how your particular cancer cells can be expected to react to drugs. Your oncologist might not give you the treatment personally, but she or he will supervise a physician's assistant or nurse trained in the procedure.

Treatment philosophies can differ slightly in the uses of chemotherapy for colon cancer, so always interview your potential oncologist first. Choose someone with whom you feel confident and one who has experience with colon and rectal cancer. Ask your doctor for some stories about how other patients helped manage their chemotherapy, how they handled their side effects, and so on.

The most important question to ask your oncologist is, "What is the goal of treatment—to cure the cancer or to slow it down?" Also ask, "What will be the plan if the chemotherapy does not work? What if the cancer metastasizes later?" Also find out which drugs will be used, how they will be administered, and how often. Be sure to ask about the side effects.

There are over 16,000 specially trained medical oncologists in the United States. One of them is likely to be near enough for you to consult. If you want to verify that any physician you plan to consult is certified in a specialty, you can contact the American Board of Specialties (1-800-776-2378).

Most libraries have reference books that list training and board certifications of practicing specialists. Ask for the *Directory of Medical Specialists*. Physicians are listed by subspecialty, by town or city, and by where they got their medical training. This is a good way to find the names of oncologists if you do not live near a comprehensive cancer center or if you want to get a second opinion.

WHERE TO GET CHEMOTHERAPY

Doctor's offices, hospital outpatient units, cancer center clinics, and even HMO cancer units all provide for the administration of chemotherapy. But if you are looking for a chemotherapy center, be sure it has the availability of emergency equipment in case of severe drug reactions and adequate staff to treat and counsel you. Because you will spend a good deal of time in the facility, it should be a pleasant environment.

If you do not live near a major cancer center or if you live in a rural area that may not have an oncologist, you can explore other alternatives. Sometimes your family doctor can obtain the appropriate drugs and provide your course of therapy after consultation with an oncologist. If your family doctor communicates frequently with the oncologist during your course of therapy, then it is sometimes possible to give chemotherapy this way.

To find out more about medical oncologists experienced with colon cancer and information about the medical center in your area, you can call the National Cancer Institute (NCI) Hotline at 1-800-4-CANCER or your local American Cancer Society (ACS) chapter.

IF YOU TAKE OTHER MEDICATIONS

It is essential to talk with your oncologist about other medications you already take. Sometimes even the most common drugs, such as aspirin, antacids, or even vitamin supplements, can interfere with certain chemotherapy drugs. In fact, make a list, and talk it over before you begin your chemotherapy. If you are not sure of the names and doses, bring the drugs to your first visit.

Keep in mind also that during your course of chemotherapy you should never take anything—even harmless over-the-counter drugs—without first talking with your oncologist. Be sure to let your other doctors know about your chemotherapy, too. They might prescribe something for some reason as seemingly harmless as eye drops or an antibiotic for dental surgery, which could interfere with your treatment. Ask them to check with your oncologist before they prescribe any drugs for you.

HOW CHEMOTHERAPY IS ADMINISTERED

For colon cancer, chemotherapy treatment is most commonly given by intravenous injection and administered weekly in your oncologist's office, but this varies. Generally, after you are examined and your blood is tested, a specially trained nurse or physician's assistant injects the medication directly into the vein (intravenous) in your arm or the back of your hand.

In addition to intravenous administration, some chemotherapy can also be intramuscular (IM), oral (PO or OS), or subcutaneous (SC—under the skin). Sometimes, a central venous access—portocath, or peripherally inserted central catheter (PIC)—is implanted in a patient's body so that drugs can easily be introduced through catheters that deliver drugs directly to the bloodstream. This might be done to allow the medication to go directly into a larger vein in the body, rather than the smaller hand or arm veins. Some physicians find this method more effective. A port might also be used for patients with weak veins or for those who cannot tolerate injections. These access ports are implanted in a minor outpatient surgical procedure and are removed by a surgeon when your chemotherapy is ended. There are several different types of ports, so ask your doctor if you are a candidate for this type procedure.

For Duke's Stage C colon cancer, chemotherapy with 5-FU and levamisole normally begins three to five weeks after surgery. This can vary in dosage amount, technique of administration, and length of time, for example, 5-FU might be given by intravenous injection daily, Monday through Friday, for four weeks, then weekly for 48 weeks starting at day 28. Levamisole might be given orally for three days every two weeks for one year.

You will feel the side effects of chemotherapy most strongly for the first day or two after you receive your dose. Most commonly, this is nausea and loss of appetite, but it will taper off. That is why the chemotherapy doses are cyclical. This gives you a chance to recuperate and regenerate your normal cells before the next dose.

TREATMENT FOR METASTATIC COLON CANCER

Fewer than half of colon cancer patients eventually develop metastatic disease either at a local or distant site. The treatment of any metastatic colon cancer requires focusing on the whole body, with the goal of easing the symptoms and halting progression of the disease for as long as possible in order to maintain a decent quality of life.

Chemotherapy

Some patients might ask, "If you can't cure my colon cancer, why should I bother with chemotherapy? Why go through a year of possible nausea and hair loss and other discomforts?" Many people ask these same questions, but the goal of chemotherapy is not always to cure cancer. Sometimes the cancer might not be considered curable, but it can be controlled for a long period of time and extend a patient's life for many years. This is the same for many chronic diseases, such as diabetes or hypertension, for which people take drugs to keep the disease under control. The average patient with cancer lives at least as long as the average patient who suffers a severe heart attack.

Chemotherapy, even if it does not cure you, often increases your survival time, and enhances your general well-being. It can relieve the symptoms of cancer so you feel better. This can add to your quality of life, despite some temporary side effects. Your oncologist's philosophy about treating advanced cancer can be of immense importance to you. Some oncologists are very aggressive about administering chemotherapy, even if the chance of cure is small or nonexistent. Others believe that withdrawing the therapy and looking after the patient's comfort are more important. It is vital for you and your doctor to talk openly and honestly about treatment.

113

If colon cancer has metastasized elsewhere, treatment depends on where the disease is showing symptoms—in the liver, bones, or lungs—and on the time span between the first diagnosis and metastatic development. Whereas surgical removal of an isolated metastasized lesion has proven successful, chemotherapy choices are fewer once you have already been treated with it. Studies are underway with infusing chemotherapy drugs directly into the colon or into the liver to concentrate the chemotherapy to the target organ involved in the metastatic disease. This technique attempts to deliver a high dose of medication to the tumor while minimizing systemic side effects.

Hepatic Artery Perfusion

The liver is the most frequent site of metastatic colon cancer. Although isolated lesions can be surgically removed successfully from the liver, more widespread disease cannot. In that case, chemotherapy can be infused directly into the liver. Hepatic artery perfusion of chemotherapy has been used for a number of years with some success. *Perfusion* is a method of forcing a fluid through an organ via blood vessels, whereas infusion is the slow, continuous introduction of drugs into a vein.

Most of the blood flow to the liver metastases comes from the hepatic artery, the main blood supply from the heart. Attempts have been made to intensify cytotoxic therapy to the liver while limiting overall toxicity to the system by administering the drug through the hepatic artery (intrahepatic chemotherapy), via a port implanted into the patient's body. According to one clinical study, this access-port method was responsible for complete disappearance of tumor in 15 percent of patients. In 39 percent of the patients, tumor size was reduced by half; and in another 21 percent of the patients studied, tumors shrank by 25 percent. Systemic drug toxicity was minimized with this artery perfusion chemotherapy, but not without damage to the healthy tissue.

Studies are underway to introduce anticancer drugs directly into the abdomen through a thin tube. This is intraperitoneal chemotherapy, not yet in general use.

Immunotherapy

This treatment is designed to help the body's own immune system attack and destroy cancer cells. It uses agents made in a patient's own body or in the laboratory to direct the body's own defenses against disease. It is sometimes called *biological response modifier* (BRM). Side effects vary widely but can include flulike symptoms such as fever, weakness, and chills, as well as nausea, vomiting, and diarrhea. Patients might also develop a rash.

Immunotherapy can be combined with chemotherapy right now, but this is not in wide use. New types of immunotherapy are being used in clinical trials of colon and rectal cancer patients.

IS A CLINICAL TRIAL RIGHT FOR YOU?

All drugs used to combat disease in humans go through many levels of testing before they are used on patients. They are tested in the laboratory (in vitro), then in animals (in vivo), then in humans in special controlled studies of volunteer patients. These are clinical studies. Usually patients with advanced cancer who could benefit by a drug that is on the cutting edge but still not in general use participate in these studies. Most of the drugs used in such trials are already known to be effective in fighting cancer, but not enough is known to be certain how much and for how long they should be administered for maximum effectiveness. All treatment regimens, such as the combination of 5-FU and levamisole, which is now a standard in colon cancer treatment, were once part of a clinical trial study.

If you have advanced colon or rectal cancer, you might want to consider participating in one of the nearly 100 national clinical studies that are in progress. Such trials are usually carried out by university teaching hospitals, but the patients studied are scattered around the country, usually in comprehensive cancer centers or in other teaching hospitals. The purpose of the studies is to find out how effective a new treatment is, so a number of patients are treated and followed with surveillance for a certain number of years.

Your medical oncologist and The National Cancer Institute can tell you which clinical trials are available for colon cancer patients. If you are a good candidate and would benefit by being part of a trial, your doctor will explain what the drugs will accomplish and how the benefit can be expected to exceed the risk of treatment. To be part of a controlled study like this, you would need to give your signed consent to take the drug in a hospital or clinic setting or in a physician's office with special rigid standards of monitoring and record keeping. Other patients in other cities with similar prognoses might be part of the same careful observation and reporting.

You are a good candidate for participation in a clinical trial if you are not burdened with additional medical problems and if you are highly motivated to undergo unproven treatment. You also need to be able to get to the university medical centers, which are often located in large cities. In general, younger patients fit the bill.

If you do join a clinical trial, do not consider yourself a guinea pig. Consider yourself fortunate to have the newest and possibly most effective drug combinations available to you. Like most opportunities in life, there is risk; but if you discuss these risks thoughtfully with your doctor—and possibly get a second opinion—you should be able to make an informed decision. If you do participate in a clinical study, it is essential that you feel trust and confidence in your doctor and the care you will get.

WHAT YOU SHOULD KNOW ABOUT CLINICAL TRIALS

Before you can make up your mind about joining a clinical trial, there are many things to know. Most important, you want to know if the physicians running the study are going to provide you with care the same way your own doctor would, or if they will be simply supervising your treatment. Here are some things to consider before making up your mind.

- **Who will care for you?** Ask the physicians who are using protocol chemotherapy who will be taking care of you. Will it be oncology fellows (young physicians in training for the subspecialty of oncology)? Will specially trained nurses, nurse practitioners, or physician's assistants be utilized? These are sometimes the people who actually give you chemotherapy.

- **Whom do you call with a question?** Who answers the phone at night or on weekends when you have a problem? You very much need to know with whom you can talk about a problem or a question so you do not feel isolated.
- **How exactly do you fit into the protocol?** What is it about your case that makes you eligible? All the aspects of your case—your age, lifestyle, genetic makeup, and health history—are considered. You should understand your role in the study and what about you is unique.
- **What if you are not happy and want to drop out?** Will you continue to get treatment or will you have to go elsewhere? Are you legally bound to continue?
- **What will be the relationship between the oncologist and your primary care physician?** You need to know that these two physicians are communicating with each other. Will they be speaking by phone or sending operative reports by fax or E-mail?
- **Does your medical insurance cover all the costs?** While the medications used in your treatment might be free to you as a participant through research grants or from drug companies, that is not the only cost consideration. The procedure itself and other costs of therapy might not be covered. Particular investigational protocols and experimental treatments are often not covered by insurance. However, this tends to be decided on an individual basis, depending upon the particular study and your particular insurance carrier.

The National Cancer Institute Hotline (1-800-4-CANCER) can provide you with the latest information about where these trials are taking place and what the qualifications are. Ask for the Community Clinical Oncology Program list of 75 medical centers in 34 states selected by NCI to participate in the newest chemotherapy protocols.

PREPARING YOURSELF FOR CHEMOTHERAPY

Naturally, you will not know precisely how chemotherapy will make you feel until you begin treatment, but it is wise to consider that there will be some disruption to your lifestyle during the treatment year. Assume you will feel some discomfort the first day or two following your treatment. So plan ahead as best you can.

Whether or not you continue to work is really up to you and will depend on how much and what kind of chemotherapy you are getting. If you feel up to it, then by all means continue working. Most people do. After all, there are not many people who can take a year off! But you will be tired for a day or two right after treatment. If you can, schedule your chemotherapy treatments late in the day or on Friday so you have the evening or the weekend to rest.

Use a calendar to plan your life around your treatment cycles for months at a time. This way you will know when you might be too nauseous to attend a dinner party or an important business meeting. By planning ahead, you can be at your best and enjoy yourself, and even eat what you like. Chemotherapy can be somewhat flexible, so, if you travel, you can either reschedule treatments or arrange to get them at a chemotherapy center where you will be traveling. Ask your oncologist about this.

You might also want to adjust your work schedule. Some employers are required by federal and state law to allow you to work a flexible or part-time schedule. (For information about such laws and other job or work-related considerations, see Chapter 17.)

MONITORING YOUR CHEMOTHERAPY

Your chemotherapist knows if your treatment is working by monitoring your progress with blood tests each time you come in for treatment and by talking with you about your health. During treatment, your oncologist might also check your weight and blood pressure. Your blood is tested for a variety of indicators to see if the chemotherapy is working and to monitor for possible toxicity. There really is nothing more to monitor, other than your possible side effects from chemotherapy. You see the results by your continued survival and lack of recurrence.

Ask your oncologist what the blood tests are showing, especially the blood tumor markers such as the carcinoembryonic antigen (CEA) assay. As mentioned earlier, the CEA is an important gauge in watching for the return of any cancer cells. It is valuable in serial monitoring. There are new markers, such as an assay called CA19-9, that also might be of value in monitoring for liver metastasis. Ask your oncologist which tests are used.

A complete blood count (CBC) to monitor white cells, red cells, and platelets during your treatment is vital. About three weeks after you start the cycle of chemotherapy, your blood counts might drop. If your counts become too low—particularly your white blood cells, which guard against infection—your chemotherapist will be able to warn you about an increased risk for infection. (Normal white blood cell count range is between 4,000 and 11,000.) Low platelet count would mean your blood will not clot. (Normal platelet count is between 140,000 and 400,000.)

Many physicians have equipment in their office that can process many tests quickly with one vial of your blood. Others send blood to the pathology department or a laboratory, and you must wait several days for results.

THE COST OF CHEMOTHERAPY

The cost of chemotherapy depends on the drugs, the dosage you are getting, and the place where you are getting your treatments. The cost is usually billed by the cycle, that is, a total for each 28-day period. This could amount to more than $1,000 per cycle. The fee for treatment includes not only the cost of drugs, but doctor visits and all the laboratory tests throughout your treatment, as well as other medications. All of this—and a wig if you need one—is generally included in health insurance coverage. If your insurance does not cover this or if you have no insurance, some of the drug companies provide free drugs for treatment to qualified patients who cannot afford to pay.

Ask your chemotherapist about the *Directory of Prescription Drug Indigent Programs,* which can help locate drugs at low or no cost. This directory is published by the Pharmaceutical Manufacturer's Association in Washington, D.C.

With so many different health care plans, it is vital to check with your oncologist about his or her participation in these plans. Some plans will not pay for treatment unless the oncologist is a member of the plan. Some closed plans, like HMOs, might limit your choice of oncologist. Many physicians will adjust their fees and work with you so that you can pay less or pay in installments.

If you are required to pay for the chemotherapy drugs yourself, pay attention to the cost. Ask oncology nurses, social workers, and health care agencies for information about fairly priced medications. A telephone survey to compare prices will help save money. Compare prices in chain and nonchain pharmacies. Many people buy without doing this. Chains are not necessarily the cheapest. If you are a union member, check with your union office. Although you probably will not have to actually purchase the drugs, you want to be sure you are getting the best price.

The National Cancer Institute (NCI) also has a booklet called *Chemotherapy and You: A Guide to Self-Help during Treatment.* This booklet explains chemotherapy and addresses problems and concerns of patients undergoing this treatment. The NCI also publishes booklets with hints for eating during chemotherapy, and other helpful booklets. Most are available in English and Spanish.

To learn how to obtain the booklet and for the latest information on chemotherapy drugs, call the NCI hotline at 1-800-4-CANCER. They have the PDQ data base with the latest information on new drugs.

Your local chapter of the American Cancer Society (ACS) should have the latest information on drugs. Call 1-800-ACS-2345.

Cancer Care might be able to help with the financial burdens of treatment. Call them at 1-800-813-HOPE (4673).

The appendices at the end of this book list numbers to call for more information about chemotherapy and how to pay for treatment.

12

COPING WITH THE
SIDE EFFECTS OF
CHEMOTHERAPY

E very patient is unique, and it is impossible to know exactly how you will be affected by chemotherapy, but most side effects of chemotherapy are temporary and tolerable. And many are reversible. There is absolutely no relationship between the effectiveness of the drugs and the extent of your side effects. The same drug can cause frequent vomiting in one person and can cause only a vague feeling of nausea or no symptoms at all in another patient. It is important to talk about your symptoms with your doctor because it is often possible to reverse some of the symptoms.

The most common side effect during chemotherapy for colon cancer is mild nausea. Perhaps one-quarter of all patients experience diarrhea, and those with sensitive skin might also have some reaction to skin and nails. Hair loss is not common with this chemotherapy, but we have included discussions of all possible side effects.

An extremely rare side effect, seen in only a fraction of patients receiving chemotherapy, is a neurological reaction that can cause mental confusion or problems in walking and moving. However, this effect is so rare that most oncologists have never observed it in any of their patients.

FOR GASTROINTESTINAL PROBLEMS

The gastrointestinal problems created by cytotoxic drugs are usually the most troublesome side effects. You cannot eat because you are nauseous, and the smell of food only makes it worse. Even food you once loved can turn your stomach. But you must eat to keep up your strength and restore the healthy cells that are being knocked out by your chemotherapy. Sores in your mouth make it difficult to swallow. The intensity of your reaction to chemotherapy is impossible to predict. But assuming you will feel sick part of the time, there are some ways to get through it.

Ask your oncologist if there are medications to help the nausea. Sometimes this can be given intravenously along with your chemotherapy so you do not get nauseous. If you are too nauseous to keep down oral drugs, some medications are available as rectal suppositories. Take these *before* the symptoms strike. Some physicians can even legally prescribe a derivative of marijuana in pill form that is frequently used to combat nausea during chemotherapy. If your symptoms are really severe, your doctor can prescribe a sedative so you can relax or sleep through the most difficult period.

Some patients have found hypnosis, biofeedback, and relaxation techniques useful. Some have learned a technique called visualization: They visualize the cytotoxic drugs killing their cancer cells. Whether or not this works for you naturally depends on your temperament and personality, but many patients have "psyched" themselves to make this kind of technique work. (There is more about this in Chapter 13.)

Remember that the side effects are strongest right after you get your treatment. You will feel better in a couple of days and gradually improve until you get the next dose. And the cycle begins again. But in the meanwhile, to keep your cells regenerating, you must eat. Your chemotherapy regimen might last a year! Some patients end up gaining a considerable amount of weight during the year of chemotherapy. Although they are too sick to eat right after each treatment, a few days later they are ravenous and eat so much that they gain weight.

However, do not worry about weight during chemotherapy. This will only add more emotional pressure. Do what works for you to get through treatment. Later, when the chemotherapy is completed, you can get back into shape. Meanwhile, here are hints for coping with side effects.

Nausea and Poor Appetite

If medications to prevent nausea do not work and you still feel sick or unable to eat, **try these:**

- Eat frequent, smaller meals.
- Try sips of water first, then a little more.
- Eat only one bite of something until you are gradually able to eat more.
- Chew your food well.
- Eat room-temperature food—their odors are less intense.
- Suck on hard candies. Jelly beans and dried candied ginger also help.
- Snack every hour to get the calories you need. Carry plain crackers or dried fruit with you.
- High-calorie drinks, such as milk shakes and breakfast drinks, can provide nourishment more easily than a meal.
- Keep your body well hydrated by drinking plenty of fluids, at least eight 8-ounce glasses of water and juices every day. This is tough if you are nauseated, but take small sips. Try clear broth to get the fluid and some nutrition at the same time.
- Eat ice cream! As a high-fat food, it has more than twice as many calories per gram as protein and carbohydrates. When chemotherapy is finished, you can work on that low-fat, high-fiber diet. Right now you want to concentrate on *not* losing weight.
- Eat meat, fish, and dairy products to get high protein to help repair your damaged normal cells.
- Breathe deeply and slowly when you feel nauseated.
- Wear loose clothing.
- You can get more help by reading the National Cancer Institute's (NCI) helpful booklet *Eating Hints: Recipes and Tips for Better Nutrition during Cancer Treatment.*

To prevent or lessen nausea, you should **avoid these:**

- Alcohol.
- Big meals.
- Carbonated beverages.
- Sweet, fried, or fatty foods.
- Lying down right after you eat.

Diarrhea

If diarrhea persists for more than 24 hours or if you are getting painful cramps, let your doctor know. There might be medications to help ease this condition. Otherwise, **try these:**

- Drink plenty of fluids such as water, apple juice, weak tea, or flat ginger ale.
- The BRAT diet—banana, rice, applesauce, toast—might work.
- Eat low-fiber foods, like white bread, eggs, ripe bananas, cottage cheese, yogurt, mashed potatoes, pureed vegetables, or fish and poultry without skin.

Avoid these:

- Raw vegetables and other high-fiber foods like beans, nuts, whole grain breads, and cereals.
- Greasy or highly spiced foods and all fried foods.
- Milk products, if these seem to make it worse.
- Tea, coffee, alcohol, and sweets.

Constipation

Constipation can be caused not so much by the chemotherapy but by other medications such as pain killers, or it can be caused by the lack of exercise when you are not feeling well. Ask your doctor if you should take any medications for this. Otherwise, **try these:**

- Drink warm and hot fluids such as coffee, tea, or soup to get things moving.
- Eat high-fiber foods like raw vegetables, fresh and dried fruits, and whole grain breads and cereals.

- Take a natural stool softener, such as Metamucil, to help maintain regularity.
- Exercise if you can—walking is good.

IF YOU HAVE MOUTH SORES

Gently brush your teeth with a very soft brush after each meal. Use a cotton swab if your toothbrush hurts. But keep your mouth as clean as possible to prevent infection. Before you rinse your mouth with commercial mouthwashes which may further irritate your mouth, ask your doctor to recommend one. Here is a simple mouth wash you can make at home to ease the sores and help keep your mouth clean.

Mouthwash

1 teaspoon of salt
1 teaspoon of baking soda
1 quart of warm water

Mix ingredients together, and rinse your mouth with it several times during the day to soothe the delicate tissue inside your mouth and to remove bacteria.

If sores are so painful you cannot eat, ask your doctor about nonprescription lozenges and sprays, such as Cepacol®, to numb your mouth and throat so that you will be able to swallow food. Or, your doctor can prescribe Xylocaine®, a local anesthetic, and Benadryl®, which you can add to the mouthwash with these changes: Boil the water and salt first, and, when that mixture is cool, then add the baking soda plus 3 tablespoons of viscous Xylocaine and 2 tablespoons of Benadryl elixir. Swish this around in your mouth. This should provide some relief. Otherwise, **try these:**

- Eat soft and soothing foods like applesauce, ice cream, or frozen yogurt.
- Drink through a straw.
- Suck on ice chips, popsicles, or sugarless candy, or chew sugarless gum.

- See your dentist for gum care, and ask for special toothpaste if your teeth and gums are sore.

  Avoid these:

- High-acid foods like citrus and spaghetti sauce.
- Very hot or very cold foods and liquids.
- Salt.
- Smoking!

EFFECTS ON SKIN AND NAILS

Ask your doctor to recommend creams or lotions to use if you develop severe dry skin, blotchy skin, a rash, or an acnelike condition that is quite common. Your skin may become pale or even discolored. Use a soft, creamy cleanser instead of soap for a while. Chemotherapy can make your skin more sensitive to irritation or sunburn, so it might be advisable to avoid direct sun. Your nails might also become brittle and break easily, or they might become ridged, so keep them short.

HAIR LOSS

Hair loss is called *alopecia*. Hair follicles of lashes, armpits, legs, scalp, beard, pubis, are made of rapidly growing cells that are the kinds of cells immediately affected by chemotherapy. Because chemotherapy affects hair follicles, the hair might break off near the scalp, and this can leave the scalp feeling tender.

Hair loss is uncommon with most chemotherapy regimens for colon cancer, but your hair might get thinner. Ask your oncologist about this. If your hair does thin out, it will be less obvious if you keep your hair short.

If your doctor tells you that a loss is certain, then get a wig before your hair falls out, unless you choose to shave your head and be bald. Some patients prefer to shave their heads rather than to watch their hair fall out gradually. Being bald may be easier for men, but some women have made a powerful and unique statement by going bald!

Try not to worry about hair loss. Your hair will grow back—everywhere—when the treatment is over. You could be surprised with a slightly different color and texture in the regrowth: Hair that was straight has been known to come back wavy or curly. Hair that was gray might grow back a darker color.

There are methods for caring for your hair as it thins. **Try these:**

- Frequent hair cuts to keep the shape.
- Very mild or baby shampoos.
- Wide tooth combs.

Avoid these:

- Shampooing too often.
- Blow dryers.
- Coloring or perming your hair (until it comes back completely).

Wigs

Wigs for men and women are widely available in specialty and department stores, as well in special stores that cater to cancer patients. A human hair wig might look great, but it will cost from $800 to $1,500, and it will need to be washed and styled. Artificial hair wigs are cheaper and easier to care for. Call around for the best prices, and ask whether there are facilities for private consultation to chemotherapy patients. The cost of a wig for use during chemotherapy is covered by medical insurance. There might be limits as to how many you can buy, however. A wig is also a tax-deductible medical expense. For more sources of wigs, **try these:**

- Your local American Cancer Society (ACS) chapter should have a list of wig suppliers in your area. Some chapters have wig banks for people with limited incomes.
- Look Good, Feel Better has a program of workshops for women available in many communities to show you how to use wigs, makeup, and nails during chemotherapy. They work in cooperation with ACS.

127

- Many private companies provide literature about using wigs during chemotherapy.
- "Buyer's Guide to Wigs and Hairpieces" is a two-page summary available from Ruth Weintraub Co., Inc., 420 Madison Avenue, New York, NY 10017, 1-212-838-1333.
- A color catalogue of wigs for medical purposes is available from Jacques Darcel, 50 West 57th Street, New York, NY 10019, 1-800-445-1897.

THE DIFFERENCE BETWEEN FATIGUE AND ANEMIA

Chemotherapy will make you feel tired simply because your body is under attack by the medication. Don't fight it and don't try to tackle a normal schedule if you are not up to it. Rest when you feel tired. If you also feel weak or dizzy and have chills and shortness of breath, you might be anemic. Your bone marrow's ability to make the red blood cells that carry oxygen around your body might be hampered by chemotherapy, so you could become anemic. If you feel dizzy, your doctor needs to know about this. In the meantime, **try these:**

- Rest often.
- Ask family and friends for help when you need it.
- Eat iron-rich foods like green leafy vegetables, raisins, and red meats.
- Get up slowly from a reclining position to prevent dizziness.
- Take a multivitamin with iron. Chewable children's vitamins are easier to tolerate if you are nauseous. Ask your pharmacist about this.

GUARDING AGAINST INFECTION

Infection is more likely because your white blood cells are being devastated during chemotherapy. These are the cells that fight infection, and if they are wiped out by chemotherapy or too low when the next cycle of chemotherapy is to start, then your treatment could be postponed until these cells regenerate. You do not need to avoid living a normal life. You just need to be aware that you might be more susceptible to infection. For example, there is no reason to avoid the company of your children or grandchildren, but if they have colds, be aware of some risk. If you suspect infection, call your doctor. You might need antibiotics. Otherwise, **try these:**

- Take especially good care of your teeth because your teeth and gums are very susceptible to infections because of the amount of bacteria in the mouth.
- Wash your hands often.
- Clean cuts and bruises immediately with antiseptic, warm water, and soap.

Avoid these:

- People who are sick with colds or flu or other communicable diseases.
- Crowds.

EFFECT ON SEXUALITY

Your sex drive might not be up to par during your course of chemotherapy, but always keep in mind that it is only temporary. This is like everything else in your life now. If you feel up to it, then do it. Affection is very important to you right now. If you and your partner can talk openly and honestly about your feelings, it will certainly help you cope with treatment. It is important to communicate with your partner—and your doctor—if you are worried about the effect of chemotherapy on your ability to enjoy sex.

As was mentioned earlier, chemotherapy can bring on an early menopause in women. Most colon cancer patients are post-menopausal, so they would not be affected. But for premenopausal women, the only difference in menopause brought on by chemotherapy is that it is an abrupt change rather than a gradual one. You must suddenly deal with an aspect of your development that you had not expected to confront yet. There could be symptoms of vaginal dryness, for example, that could inhibit the enjoyment of sex. (Read Chapter 18 for information on reversing the effects of colon cancer treatment on sexuality and for resources for more information.)

WHEN SIDE EFFECTS ARE SEVERE

Call your oncologist if any of the following occur.

- Chills and fever, cold or flu symptoms.
- Swelling or redness around the injection site.
- Profuse bleeding when you cut yourself.
- Bruising easily.
- Blood in urine or stool, black stool, or profuse diarrhea.
- Becoming anorexic.
- Mental changes.
- Dizziness or fainting.

Most patients experience very mild side effects and they go to work, travel, and lead normal lives. But always ask your doctor if you suspect a side effect is too intense or if you develop an unexpected side effect. Talk with people in your support group. This is another good reason for that network. You can compare notes about treatment and side effects.

13

NONMEDICAL AIDS
TO TREATMENT

It is always easier to get through a difficult time if you have a warm and supportive network of family and friends or if you belong to a sympathetic support group. The weeks and months after diagnosis and treatment can cause you to be afraid and anxious. You might have all kinds of preconceived notions about what colon cancer treatment is and what is going to happen to you. Various procedures, tests, surgery, and talks with doctors can prompt a great deal of anxiety. As you become more familiar with the treatment routine, your anxiety will diminish. Nevertheless, the diagnosis and treatment, both short- and long-term, can compromise your self esteem and can disrupt your family and schedule.

EMOTIONAL AND PRACTICAL SUPPORT
FROM FAMILY AND FRIENDS

If you already have a warm and loving circle of family and friends, you are in luck. But face it, your cancer can cause them stress, too, and put up road blocks in communication. Sometimes people will not know what to say or do, so they often say and do nothing for fear of making you feel worse. It is always a good idea to be precise and specific. Explain to your family exactly what your surgery and recuperation means. Share with them what you have learned.

131

Try to communicate your feelings and needs. If you want their help or moral support, ask for it. You cannot expect those who love you to read your mind and automatically provide all kinds of comfort and support. It is better to ask. For instance, once you are home, you might need some help around the house or with your work. Or you might not feel up to cooking and would appreciate having someone bring you meals or cook for you. Sometimes you might just want someone to hang out with you.

HOME HEALTHCARE WORKERS

You might want to engage a home healthcare worker for the first week or so after the hospital, especially if you live alone, have complications from surgery, or have additional medical problems with which to cope. Sometimes this is helpful for older patients or for those who have an ill spouse at home who would not be able to help them. This can be arranged through your hospital social work department or the home healthcare department.

Health care is more inclined to include this coverage because it keeps the patient out of the hospital, which costs a great deal more. A home healthcare nurse can come to check your vital signs and change your dressings each day for a week, then perhaps visit less often. With this kind of professional help, you can also relieve some anxiety and reinforce your training about your new condition, such as adapting to a colostomy.

Ask about this while you are at the hospital and find out if you are eligible. This is a very gray area in terms of medical insurance coverage, too. If your doctor says you require wound care or you need help with taking your medications or with ostomy appliances, antibiotics, or bed sores, then your medical insurance might cover the cost. There could be limitations, however, such as the number of visits by a nurse or home healthcare aide that will be covered.

If a healthcare worker will be coming to see you for a period of time, perhaps several weeks, it is important to develop a rapport with that person. He or she will be spending time with you, helping you, and seeing you at your most vulnerable. If you have made your best effort, but you do not like this particular healthcare worker, call your hospital or home healthcare agency and ask them to send someone else.

SUPPORT GROUPS

This is not the time to hide away by yourself. Even a loving family and friends are not always enough. You need to talk with other people who know what it is like to have colon or rectal cancer or to live with a colostomy. Even if you are coping well, you might enjoy the camaraderie of a group, and you could also be a good role model for another person.

Cancer support groups help you feel less anxious, less depressed, less afraid, and thus you might experience less pain. These groups can offer one of the best ways to get yourself through a rough time, as well as a place where you can feel safe and secure, where everybody understands what you are going through. You do not have to hide your fears or pretend everything is all right. You can express your anger, shed your tears, and laugh at life's ironies.

Support groups help you through this time by letting you know how others cope with their jobs, families, and friends who do not know what to say or do. You don't have to prove how brave you are. Don't do it alone! There is no substitute for the emotional bond that develops among people in a good cancer support group.

There are support groups for all types of cancer survivors and some for particular cancers. Ask the nurses and doctors at your treatment center if there is one just for colon cancer. And if you find that you do not identify with people in one group or if the people are too negative for your sensibility, then try to find another one. You should be able to find a group that is the right one for you.

It would be unusual if there was not some cancer support group in your community, but look for one that is just for colon cancer. Call your local ACS chapter for information on cancer survivor groups. You can also ask at your hospital social work department, or you can call the Cancer Information Center at the NCI for the booklet *Taking Time: Support for People with Cancer and the People Who Care about Them*. And the National Coalition for Cancer Survivorship publishes a periodic newsletter. (See Appendix 1 for the address.)

If there are no support groups in your area, think about starting one. This takes a lot of work, but it can be rewarding.

PRIVATE COUNSELING

If you are unable or unwilling or too shy to participate in a support group to get you through the trauma of treatment, you might feel more comfortable talking privately with a psychologist or psychiatrist for short-term counseling. There is a newly developing therapeutic specialty called psycho-oncology, and you might be able to locate a therapist who specializes in the emotional aspects of cancer. Many comprehensive cancer treatment centers now routinely offer this service.

There has been more recognition by the healthcare establishment over the past decade that cancer patients have unique emotional needs as well as potential psychological problems to address. They need to adjust not only to the illness, but to how it interacts with other emotional problems, their culture, age, or sex. And they need to cope with the impact on their families.

More often than not, short-term counseling—once or twice a week for a few weeks—is all that is needed to get you through the therapeutic process. Therapy can be one-on-one with your therapist, or you can go with your spouse or partner or family member. Some of these resources may be able to help you locate someone:

- The American Medical Association.
- The American Psychiatric Association.
- Your local hospital oncology or psychiatry department, social worker, or patient services representative.

STRESS REDUCTION TECHNIQUES

Some cancer centers offer behavioral therapy, such as visualization, biofeedback, and relaxation techniques, that can help you cope and feel in control of your treatment and recovery. Acupuncture, hypnosis, and Zen meditation are also available, but here are some techniques that are recognized by health professionals as the most effective.

- **Biofeedback** is a technique of learning to monitor your own muscle tension and to intervene to relax that tension. Skin elec-

134

trodes monitor subtle changes in temperature, muscle, perspiration, blood pressure, heart rate, and rhythm. By observing what your muscles are doing—signals from the electrodes form graphs on a video screen—you can learn to intervene and change them. It can also help you relax before treatments and reduce the symptoms of nausea and vomiting caused by chemotherapy. Most large hospital psychiatry departments and an increasing number of cancer centers have a biofeedback therapist on staff. Medical insurance often covers this therapy.

- **Visualization** is also known as guided imagery, and with some instruction and training, a patient can achieve a relaxed state by imagining they are in a more pleasant situation, such as lying on a beach or floating in an expanse of calm water. Cancer patients are often helped to imagine their cancer cells being knocked out by their chemotherapy drugs, for example. By putting themselves into this kind of state before or during their chemotherapy treatments, they can often make the experience more pleasant and feel more positive that their treatment is succeeding. Patients can also visualize themselves free of pain or stress, and this can be an effective way to meet a stressful challenge such as cancer treatment.

- **Meditation** has been practiced by people for centuries to achieve a higher level of consciousness, thus ridding their psyches of stress. More and more health professionals recommend it as a way to manage stress and pain. There are no hard and fast rules on how to meditate. Not everyone needs to sit on the floor for hours in the lotus position, which may be difficult to achieve if you are recovering from surgery. The most important aspect is to close your eyes, breath in and out slowly and calmly, and concentrate on that breathing, letting all thoughts fall away. There are many books and videos on the market that can help you learn meditation techniques and how to achieve a relaxed and tranquil state of mind.

There is a great deal available today to aid you on your voyage through cancer treatment. Take advantage of everything that is available to you to make your cancer treatment more positive and comfortable.

PART III

RECOVERY

14

TAKING CHARGE
OF YOUR
FOLLOW-UP CARE

Naturally, you do not want a recurrence of colon or rectal cancer, but you must look for it always by going in for your regular checkups and screenings. These will make you apprehensive. This is normal. Tell yourself if you find anything such as another polyp, it will be curable because it was detected early. Denial is the worst thing. By failing to watch and follow up you are canceling out all you have been through. This is a double-edged sword in a way. You want to recover and forget about cancer, to get on with your life. But at the same time, you will always be watching for recurrence now that you are at greater risk for colon cancer.

Astute surveillance is necessary after any cancer, even if your treatment removed all the cancer. You should have a colonoscopy from three to six months after a colectomy and again 12 months after to detect recurrences of the primary tumor and development of others. The majority of recurrence appears within two years of the initial operation. During the next two years, you will be examined about every three months. After that it will be less often, but for the rest of your life, regularly scheduled checkups, including sigmoidoscopies and/or colonoscopies, are mandatory!

SCHEDULING VISITS TO YOUR TREATMENT TEAM

Your gastroenterologist, surgeon, and medical oncologist will monitor your healing process periodically and check for possible recurrence. Who is going to coordinate all of this? If you feel most comfortable with your family doctor, then ask if he or she will help coordinate your care. But whether or not any of your doctors agrees to be an overseer, your follow-up care will not get organized and appointments will not be made unless you are in charge. It is up to you to keep each of your doctors informed about what the others are doing.

Keep track of your visits and schedules, and know when your next examination is due. Do this in a routine, business-like way, and it will be easier to handle. You will always feel anxious before your next sigmoidoscopy, colonoscopy, or blood test. Everyone does. But do not let anxiety—or the cost—prevent you from following up. The cost of follow-up care is expensive (estimated at $25,000), but it crucial to your future well-being. Most of this follow-up care is covered by medical insurance plans, but it would be a good idea to check on this in advance.

- **Your family doctor.** While other physicians are keeping tabs on your colon cancer, your overall health needs attention. An annual physical checkup should be part of your routine, and it should include digital and fecal occult blood tests and chest X rays. Other tests and lab work depend on your age and condition. Keep your family doctor well informed about your follow-up care with your colon cancer treatment team, such as colonoscopy or blood test results from your oncologist. If you do not have a family doctor or primary care physician, this would be a good time to get one.
- **Surgeon.** Your surgeon will examine your abdominal incision to be sure you are healing properly and that you are not developing a seroma (fluid under the skin) or flap necrosis (when the skin at the wound edges dies), a rare occurrence. After a year, there is generally no further need to visit your surgeon unless the disease recurs.

140

- **Gastroenterologist.** Follow-up will depend upon the procedures you have been through. If you are getting chemotherapy, your physicians might not want to do a colonoscopy until your treatment is completed. If your cancer is cured, you will probably return in a year for a colonoscopy. If there is risk of residual cancer, then you might need a colonoscopy sooner, perhaps in three or six months. If no cancer is found, then you will not need a repeat for 6 to 12 months. Then see your gastroenterologist for annual screenings for life.
- **Medical oncologist.** If you are taking chemotherapy, your medical oncologist is the primary physician monitoring the treatment of cancer. He or she will likely help coordinate the efforts of all the physicians you are seeing. Physician-to-physician communication—facilitated by you—is important. If you are receiving cytotoxic chemotherapy, your oncologist will routinely monitor your blood before and during treatment.

  Once treatment is over and your white blood cells and platelets are stable, quarterly blood counts for the first two years, then semiannual counts, might be all that is necessary to monitor your blood for evidence of metastatic disease. The CEA assay—carcinoembryonic antigen levels—are considered crucial indicators for this. If CEA levels are elevated, then more testing would be done to ascertain whether or not the disease is recurring.

  Your oncologist might also recommend CAT scans of your abdomen for metastatic deposits, if that is a threat. A lesion has to be greater than 1 to 2 centimeters to show up on the scan. Any suspicious new findings might warrant a needle biopsy.
- **Radiation oncologist.** If you had radiation therapy for rectal cancer, your radiation oncologist might want to examine you every three or six months for a year to look for any lingering redness or swelling and to monitor for recurrence. Radiation therapists tend to have a very focused view toward the patient regarding the area they have treated unless otherwise requested to do more by the oncologist. After a year, there is usually no further need to visit the radiation oncologist.

MAINTAINING VIGILANCE

Nobody knows if a cancer will recur. The odds can only be calculated based on everything learned through diagnosis and treatment. By understanding type and size of tumor, cell activity, lymph node status, and staging, it can be *estimated* that someone has a 10 percent chance of recurrence or a 65 percent chance, but this does not mean it will recur. Nor is there any guarantee that you will not have a recurrence even with a 5 percent chance.

Colon cancer is a particularly virulent form of cancer and can be very unpredictable. Recurrence can be:

- Local—reappearance at the same site (the colon).
- Regional—reappearance near the original site (lymph nodes).
- Metastatic—reappearance elsewhere in your body (liver, lungs, bone).

Your colon cancer could recur in your colon, or elsewhere in your system, a year or even decades later. Generally, five cancer-free years means you have beaten the heaviest odds. Eighty percent of recurrences happen within the first five years after initial treatment; and the other 20 percent occur years later.

It is estimated that about 5 percent of patients will develop a second cancer after the removal of a primary colorectal cancer. If your colon cancer was in situ and confined to the polyp, you have the lowest chance of recurrence, often less than 5 percent. Risk increases if the cancer broke out of the polyp and invaded the colon lining or wall or spread to the lymph nodes or adjoining organs.

Your pathology reports can help you understand this. Many reports summarize the findings and list a recurrence factor as a percentage. Go over these reports with your doctors so you understand the information.

With regular follow-up care, you are maintaining vigilance. Try not to become obsessed with looking for a new cancer, but do pay attention to signals from your body. Call your doctor if you have a persistent cough, gastrointestinal problems, or unexplained loss of appetite or weight changes or if you are dizzy or have frequent headaches, jaundice, or leg weakness. Never hesitate to bring anything to your doctor's attention. That is what he or she is here for. If it is of concern, the doctor will pursue it. If it turns out not to be important, then you will feel better, and your doctor will know that you are paying attention to your health.

15

STAYING HEALTHY
AFTER
COLON CANCER

R eading the health columns in the newspapers and watching reports on television can cause a lot of confusion about what is and is not good for us. It seems to change from one day to the next. There are no hard and fast rules about diet and exercise, but common sense suggests that the best course is to eat well-balanced meals with plenty of fresh fruits and vegetables, to exercise regularly, and to get plenty of rest.

It cannot be said definitely that a person who eats lots of animal fat and no fiber, unless they change their diet, will get colon cancer. Nor can it be said for sure that every person who smokes will get lung cancer. However, people with such obviously poor habits do have the odds stacked against them. A change of diet is not as dramatically therapeutic against colon cancer as quitting smoking would be in preventing lung cancer, but many more gastroenterological problems are likely in a person whose diet is loaded with animal fats and no fiber. So whether or not such poor habits cause a recurrence of colon cancer is almost beside the point.

EXERCISING THE DIGESTIVE SYSTEM

It will take a while after surgery or chemotherapy to feel like walking to the corner, never mind run a marathon, but do get moving as soon as you feel up to it. Exercise strengthens your heart and lungs and lifts your spirits. And even more important to your recovery from colon cancer, it aids digestion, helps eliminate gaseousness, and combined with balanced diet, will help keep your digestive system—and your colon—fit.

Getting Exercise

Try to make exercise directed toward muscle strength and cardiovascular fitness part of your daily routine. Walking is one of the best cardiovascular exercises. Even if you walk everyday for only half an hour, this will help you stay fit and keep your intestines functioning well. Walk as quickly as you can with your arms swinging. Start slowly, but let it become part of your life. Once your body gets used to exercising, it will crave it, and soon a good habit will develop. You need at least 20 minutes of vigorous exercise three times a week. If you do exercise for longer than 20 minutes at a time, you will start to burn off calories.

If you have access to a health club or YMCA, that is a good place to start. People of all ages and conditions participate in fitness programs these days. Treadmills, lifecycles, stairclimbers, and rowing machines are all metered to tell you how much work you are doing. The best machines for cardiovascular fitness put your large muscles in motion.

If you are still undergoing chemotherapy, ask your doctors about exercising. There are times during treatment when exercise could be harmful, for example, within 24 hours of receiving intravenous chemotherapy or if you have been nauseated or vomited in the past 24 to 36 hours. You might be dehydrated, and therefore too weak to tolerate exercise.

Controlling Weight

The most important aspect of the diet in America is eating too much. A 1996 Harris poll concluded that 74 percent of Americans are overweight. Few people need more than 2,000 calories a day, yet 3,700 calories is closer to the daily average caloric intake by Americans. Processing this much food is hard work for the digestive system.

The U.S. Census Bureau estimated that approximately 58 million adults—32 million women and 26 million men—are overweight or obese, and the number is growing. *Obese* is defined as being 20 percent above desirable weight. This number represents over one-third of the adult U.S. population. Obesity rates continue to increase, from 25 percent in 1980 to 33.4 percent in 1991.

The more food that passes through the colon, the greater the risk of colon cancer, according to the American Cancer Society (ACS). The risk increases 2.3 percent for each 100 calories per day. Indeed, some scientists have called colon cancer the disease of "overnutrition." The ACS also found that the fatter you are, the greater your risk for cancer of the breast, uterus, gallbladder, kidney, stomach, and colon. Being obese—20 percent above your ideal weight—puts you at the highest risk.

There is no magic way to lose weight. To maintain your proper weight, eat well, count calories, and exercise. To calculate the ideal weight for an adult, add five pounds to 100 for every inch of height over five feet. If you are five-foot-seven, you should weigh 135 pounds, give or take a few pounds for different bone and body structure. At six feet, you should weigh about 160.

If You Gained Weight During Your Chemotherapy

Talk with your oncologist about the best way to lose any extra weight. Some doctors recommend the Weight Watchers® program as a sane and sensible way to lose weight. It is important not to go on any crash diets or diets that are all liquid or that emphasize one particular kind of food. Those diets will affect normal body chemistry, leave your immune system at risk, and deprive you of important nutrients. The best diet is a balanced diet. Just eat smaller portions.

THE TRUTH ABOUT FIBER AND COLON CANCER

Fiber is a generic term for a wide variety of nondigestible forms of carbohydrate found in almost all vegetables, fruits, and grains. Bran is what is talked about most, and the cereal business has prospered with the "eat more bran" message. Bran is the coating of seeds and of cereal grains comprised of fibers and other substances that affect epithelial cells lining the colon. Most raw fruits and vegetables have more useful fiber than those that have been peeled, blended, cooked, or processed. Whole wheat bread has more fiber than white; an orange has more fiber than its juice.

Fiber advocates appeared as early as the nineteenth century with Sylvester Graham, who praised the properties of whole grain breads and invented the Graham cracker. He might have been thinking that there was less colon cancer in the stone age when humans ate mouse bones, horns, hair, and all kinds of unprocessed foods. In 1890, Dr. John Harvey Kellogg set up his health spa in Battle Creek, Michigan, to try out his theories about fiber. He also invented cereals like shredded wheat and granola and made a fortune with his cereal empire and his fiber message. Then something happened, and the American establishment decided that processed foods were the most healthful and ushered in the age of refinement—the age of white bread. It was not until the 1970s that the phrase *dietary fiber* was coined, and the stone-age diet came back in vogue.

It has been theorized that without sufficient fiber in the diet, food takes two to three times longer to pass through the colon, often resulting in constipation. This means harmful bacteria are hanging around in your digestive tract and leaning on your intestine walls long enough to cause trouble. Fiber is *thought* to decrease fecal transit time and to keep bacteria from becoming trapped and stagnant, thus allowing less contact between carcinogens and the colon walls. However, while increased fiber intake probably increases fecal bulk, there has been no *consistent* evidence that a high-fiber intake actually shortens the transit time of stool. For example, one study showed that a diet with 10 percent wheat bran inhibited tumor production; but if fiber was increased to 20 percent, it enhanced proliferation of cells in the colon and either had no effect on tumor production or, in one study of rats, actually increased tumor production. So too much fiber could also cause problems, although it seems unlikely anyone would consume too much.

Additional reasons that fiber is recommended is because some fiber also tends to bind substances and help them leave the body. It binds with cholesterol and bile acids, which can be implicated in cancer. Thus, fiber may reduce cholesterol levels in the blood. Fiber can also bind with iron, zinc, calcium, and other minerals and remove them from your system. Other fibers undergo a fermentation process that defuses volatile fatty bile acids. Fiber also delays the absorption of sugar so that sugar levels are better controlled.

The American diet, until recent consciousness raising, has been deficient in fiber as compared with non-Western populations. Although fiber intake is generally higher in countries where the incidence of colon cancer is low, there are many other environmental differences between developing and industrialized countries that play into this difference. Nevertheless, many physicians encourage patients to eat more fiber after they have been treated for colon cancer. It might keep the colon healthier.

A diet low in fiber can lead to chronic constipation and associated conditions such as diverticulosis. But if a low-fiber diet were a major cause of colon cancer, individuals who have diverticulosis would be at higher risk, and this does not appear to be the case.

The down side is that fiber, if you are not used to it, can cause flatulence. This is a normal reaction, so increase fiber gradually into your diet, and flatulence will subside in a few weeks.

DOES ANIMAL FAT CAUSE COLON CANCER?

The low-fat message is so popular that food companies have raced to develop low-fat and no-fat cookies, ice cream, and other products. Bold "no fat" or "low fat" labels stand out on more and more food packages.

Too much animal fat does clog the arteries and causes heart attack. But does a high-fat diet also cause colon cancer? Many medical scientists believe it does, but all the evidence is not yet in. Animal fat, such as that found in meat and butter, is said to be more harmful than vegetable fats, like olive oil, and certain fish oils. There tends to be less colon cancer in regions where fish is a big part of the diet. Also, supplements of marine fish oils were shown in some studies to lower the risk. Some believe that fish oil contains other fats that protect against colon cancer.

Studies of people who ate beef, pork, or lamb daily, compared to those who ate it less often than once a month, positively associate animal fat with colon cancer incidence. However, animal fat in dairy products—butter, cheese, and cream—was less risky because the daily consumption was lower. Fish and skinned chicken was associated with lower risk. Industrialized nations are connected with the highest meat consumption and highest rates of colon cancer. The developing countries, mostly vegetarians or fish and grain eaters, have less colon cancer.

Research indicates that a high intake of animal fat is the dietary element that is most strongly associated with the risk of colon cancer. The appearance of this cancer in Japan has increased as that nation has assumed a diet more like that of the Western world.

There have also been studies connecting cholesterol rates with colon cancer as well as heart disease. Animal fat increases bile acids and fatty-acid secretions, and patients with colon cancer have relatively high levels of these acids when compared to vegetarians. One study showed that an increase in animal fat from 62 grams to 152 grams per day produced significantly more fecal bile acid and fatty acid secretion.

In the United States, there had been an 18-year decline in the consumption of red meat, while the cholesterol police nagged about fat consumption. Red meat does have more fat and cholesterol than white meat like chicken or veal. Studies seem to indicate that Western populations, where red meat is highly consumed, have more colon cancer than vegetarian communities, such as in Africa or Asia. However, it is possible that Western populations—with more wealth—simply eat more food, period. The highest percentage of overweight people live in industrialized nations.

It is a good idea to cut the fat in your diet. Fat, like salt and sugar, is addictive. And this makes it harder to quit. It will take about three months to withdraw from fat. You might not be able to quit, cold turkey. Most American diets contain 40 percent fat, when 20 percent fat would be much healthier. When you try to curb your hunger with a carrot rather than a bowl of ice cream, your fat cells will be screaming for satisfaction. A glass of whole milk is eight times fattier than skim milk. If your diet is 2,000 calories, then you can have only 400 fat calories a day—or 44.4 grams of fat—on a 20 percent fat diet.

Make it a practice to read labels on packaged foods and to avoid those with high percentage of fat. Look for an inexpensive pocket guide to calories and fat grams available in most bookstores. Many are available free from health agencies such as the ACS and the American Heart Association.

VEGETABLES AND FRUIT

Vegetables and fruit are not only good sources of fiber and vitamins, they might contain other elements that play a role in cancer prevention. Chemists analyzing vegetables have discovered many healthful properties. Some of these vegetable compounds seem to retard the cell breakdowns that result in cancer.

But reports are contradictory. Betacarotene, the precursor of Vitamin A, is a good example. For years, it was believed that betacarotene inhibited cancer cell proliferation; but, in 1996, the conclusion of a long-term study revealed that it had no effect on cancer cells and, in fact, might have increased the incidence of cancer in some cases.

The scientific community has only just begun to study diets, and there are many things they do not know. There could be elements in vegetables that *encourage* cancer, too, although the positive benefits far outweigh any potential hazards. Naturally occurring food substances can be metabolized into mutagens. For example, bracken fern, which cattle eat (and, thus, is in beef), contains at least two carcinogens. Another potent carcinogen is a natural substance of mushrooms. If you eat five pounds of mushrooms a day, you might be pushing your risk level, but the digestive system is so complex and variable that it cannot be known for sure if these processes will take place in your body. To put it in the most simple terms, a cancer cell or mutagen can take up residence in your body, hang around, and do nothing and eventually leave of its own accord. Or it can dig in and start trouble with nearby cells.

Pesticides and fertilizers are also under scrutiny by medical researchers. The metabolic fate of toxic chemicals synthesized by plants as a defense against bugs, animals, and bacteria is extremely complex and varies greatly in every individual.

150

Variety and moderation in diet offers the best protection from the naturally occurring mutagens and carcinogens that cannot be avoided—whether they are pesticides used to grow fruits and vegetables, hormones fed to market animals, or pollutants ingested by fish. If you tried to avoid everything that might potentially cause a cell mutation, you would starve to death.

Antioxidants

Antioxidants act like the body's own nutrition police, protecting it from free radicals. While you are breathing and burning up energy, cells continuously generate hazardous waste that can set the stage for cancer. This waste is made of molecules known as free radicals. Poor nutrition leaves antioxidant levels low. Vitamins A, C, and E are all antioxidants. Good food sources of antioxidants are melons and citrus fruits, yellow and green vegetables, tomatoes, green leafy vegetables, potatoes, wheat germ, oatmeal, peanuts, and brown rice.

Garlic and broccoli are especially rich in antioxidants. In fact, the National Cancer Institute (NCI) puts garlic high on its list of foods that supply natural antioxidants. Eaten raw, garlic also stimulates immunological functions, lowers blood cholesterol, thins blood, and helps prevent embolisms.

Vitamin C and E might have preventive components, according to some studies. However, large numbers of people must be studied for long periods of time before any conclusions can be drawn about the benefit of vitamins in preventing cancer. A well-balanced diet will provide most of the vitamins you need.

Cruciferous Vegetables

Broccoli, cabbage, cauliflower, and Brussels sprouts are some of the cruciferous vegetables. They contain substances that are thought to inhibit cancer in animals, but there is still no definitive proof that they will protect humans. So there is no need to eat a pound of broccoli every day. Just include it in your meal once in a while (unless you have a colostomy and want to avoid gas-causing vegetables). Broccoli is high in fiber, too. Sulforaphane, which is also found in broccoli, appears to be an anticancer agent. This and

151

other isocyothionates found in cruciferous vegetables seem to stimulate production of protective enzymes in the body.

Genisten is an element found in soybeans and some cruciferous vegetables, which blocks angiogenesis—the growth of new blood vessels. If this could be used in treatment, it might prevent cancer cells from developing new capillaries that supply blood to tumors.

CALCIUM AND VITAMIN D

Calcium appears to have some role in the regulation of the cells lining the colon, although it is not entirely clear how this works. Diets supplemented with calcium seem to minimize bile acids. Laboratory studies have also suggested that calcium can inactivate carcinogens from fatty acids because it has an emulsifying action, much the way detergent cuts the grease in a frying pan. When calcium was added to the diet of 10 relatives of colon cancer patients, it significantly reduced the growth of colon epithelial cells. A survey of the diets of 1,954 men for 19 years also suggested that the risk of colon cancer is inversely correlated with oral intake of calcium and vitamin D. (Vitamin D aids the action of calcium by acting as its escort into the bloodstream.)

One-third of the Women's Health Initiative, a major clinical trial in the United States, is to investigate the effect of calcium and vitamin D on colon cancer. It will be many years before the results of this trial are known, but it should produce more definitive information about calcium and colon cancer. (If you want more information about this trial, call 1-800-54-WOMEN (549-6636), and you will be connected with a participating clinical center in your area.)

Calcium is not produced by the body, so adequate amounts of calcium must be present in your diet. It is present in all food groups, including dairy products, leafy green vegetables such as kale and spinach, nuts and beans, and certain seafoods such as salmon and canned sardines. It is also present in fortified orange juice and in some fortified cereals, oranges, and raw carrots.

Contradictory results have been reported by other controlled trials, it cannot be said definitively that if you take calcium supplements or drink a quart of milk a day, you will never get colon cancer.

(For more information about calcium, call the Calcium Information Center (CIC) at 1-800-321-2681. The CIC, which sponsors the CIC Information Line, is a component of the Clinical Nutrition Research Units of The New York Hospital Cornell Medical Center and Memorial Sloan-Kettering Cancer Center, and Oregon Health Sciences University. The CIC provides informational materials about calcium nutrition and specific health conditions, and they will answer individual telephone inquiries.)

AN ASPIRIN A DAY?

In 1991, an ACS survey of more than 660,000 people revealed a significant reduction in colon cancer deaths among people who used aspirin more than 16 times a month. But even more impressive, the aspirin apparently reduces about 40 percent of the deaths from cancer of the rectum, esophagus, and stomach. The protection is greatest among those who used it for more than 10 years. A Harvard study of female nurses found the risk of colon cancer dropped when they took as few as four to six aspirin a week. But the benefits do not start for at least a decade. The same findings are assumed to apply to men.

Researchers believe aspirin works only on the earliest stage of the colon cancer. They believe it stops the growth of polyps (the number and size of polyps) in the colon that, over time, might become cancerous. Just how it works is still unclear. It might be the aspirin's ability to block production of prostaglandins, certain fatty acids, which might regulate cell growth.

Many studies show that regular aspirin users have less colon cancer. One aspirin every other day for 20 years is said to cut the risk of colon cancer nearly in half. Some doctors routinely recommend aspirin to patients over 50 to cut the risk of heart disease, an already well-established benefit of aspirin. However, any amount of aspirin in certain individuals can cause blood loss, usually from the stomach lining, and that will appear in the stool. (Note: *Always consult your physician before using any medications, no matter how beneficial they might seem.*)

16

LIVING WITH A COLOSTOMY

There are more than one million "ostomates" in the United States and Canada. Ostomates are people with ostomies—ileostomy, urostomy, colostomy. You might know one without knowing it. They work, play, enjoy life just as they did before their surgery. Some are famous professional athletes, politicians, and entertainers. If you have joined the ranks of ostomates, there is no reason you cannot lead a perfectly normal and active life—you can work, swim, make love, and feel good about yourself.

In the past, a patient stayed in the hospital after a colostomy for about three weeks until doctors were certain the patient would be okay on his or her own. Now, the emphasis is on home care and patient responsibility. This means arranging for a home healthcare nurse who comes daily for at least one week to check vital signs, check the healing process, and continue teaching the patient how to manage life with a colostomy. Gradually, the visits are cut back as the patient and family assume the responsibility.

Wearing "the bag" is not as offensive as it used to be, when colostomy appliances were larger and made of rubber and did not keep odors from escaping. Now, these receptacles for disposing of wastes are pouches made of lightweight plastic in a more streamlined design and have charcoal filtering devices to eliminate odor. You can even learn how to self-irrigate your colon so that you do not need to wear the appliance at all.

CARE OF THE STOMA

For the four to eight weeks following surgery, the stoma will probably shrink. There is no feeling in the stoma. It cannot sense pain or the passage of waste. However, it is made of sensitive flesh with blood vessels that can bleed if irritated.

The stoma itself does not need to be cleaned because it is made of body tissue that is normally in contact with waste substances, but it might bleed slightly when you change the appliance or clean the surrounding skin.

The most common problem that ostomates have is leakage of stool around the stoma. Stool can irritate the skin around the stoma, so make sure your appliance fits properly and adheres well so it does not leak. Change it as often as recommended. Measure your stoma frequently to be sure the appliance you use is the proper size. A prickly-heat type rash may develop under the pouch and for this an antifungal ointment is applied. Some people become allergic to the pouches or patches or adhesives after many years and change brands.

Gently clean the skin surrounding the stoma each time you remove the appliance. Use only mild soap and lots of water. Don't use creams or powders unless they are recommended by your doctor or ET nurse. Never rub your skin dry. Just pat it gently.

Contact your surgeon or ET nurse if your stoma bleeds excessively, has a black color, is swollen or recedes, or has a strong, lasting odor. Also call attention to any unusual changes in body wastes or to minor skin irritations that last more than a few days. Any problem can become severe or cause pain.

USING COLOSTOMY APPLIANCES

Wearing a colostomy pouch is neither as difficult nor as unpleasant to live with as you probably imagine. Today's appliances are not bulky and do not show under even the most stylish, form-fitting clothing on men or women. A pouch attaches to the stoma cap and hangs down against the lower left side of your abdomen. It lies flat against your body, but you can pick a comfortable spot to wear it so you can see it. Whatever clothing you wore before your colostomy, you can wear now with very few exceptions. Pouches are odor-free and come in a variety of disposable and reusable types to fit your lifestyle. You are fitted for an appliance just as you are fitted for shoes or eyeglasses.

In addition to a cap and pouch, your colostomy appliance kit comes with coordinated equipment. Read all the literature that comes with your appliance and coordinated equipment. Get to know your appliance well. You will have a belt, closure tape, skin barrier, and deodorant. These items are available through supply houses, by mail order, and in drug stores. Ostomy nurses report that it is best to buy appliances directly from a mail order source or local surgical supply house in order to assure reliable service. Having your pharmacist order them for you can cause delays, or you will be dealing with someone who is not totally familiar with the appliances. Choose appliances that are leakproof, odorless, durable, lightweight, easy to use, comfortable, nonirritating to the skin, and affordable.

Most two-piece reusable colostomy bags—wafer and pouch—cost about $6 or $7 by mail order or from a surgical supply house. Insurance covers 80 percent of the cost and often you can arrange for the supply house to bill you only for the remaining 20 percent. Medicare covers the cost of 10 sets a month but will not pay for the disposable appliances unless you have a strong medical reason why they are necessary.

Adapting to a New Personal Routine

It will take some adjusting to get used to going to the bathroom in a new way. And you might find yourself spending more time in the bathroom until you become proficient managing your ostomy. It may seem frustrating at first, but be patient. Eventually, this will be only a minor inconvenience.

Here are some hints to make the process as easy as possible.

- Always wash your hands before removing or changing the appliance.
- Empty the pouch when it is one-third full and before you go to bed.

- Keep all of your appliance equipment and refills within easy reach when you go to the bathroom.
- Sit on the toilet seat or a chair and empty your appliance into the toilet.
- Hold a piece of gauze or tissue over your stoma to prevent leakage as you remove your appliance.
- When you put on your appliance, center it carefully over your stoma.
- Stand up and use a mirror or paper guide strip to help center the appliance.

The Self-Irrigation Procedure

Some ostomates do not need to wear the pouch at all because they are able to regulate their digestive systems and self-irrigate. Stool can be released directly into the toilet through a plastic sleeve attached to the stoma.

To irrigate your colon, you insert a tube into your stoma and instill about a quart of water to flush out your colon. It is similar to an enema. This way you can schedule your bowel movements. When that is done, you then simply wear a cap over your stoma, and you are ready to meet your day without worry about the pouch. Learning this procedure might take some time. In order to feel confident that there will be no accidents, you need to structure your diet so you are able to know when self-irrigation will be effective. This may take some experimenting with what you eat and when you eat. If you are still undergoing chemotherapy or radiation therapy, hold off on self-irrigation. Once the course of therapy is ended, you will be able to tackle this.

Dealing with Gas and Odors

Most people would be embarrassed and humiliated to pass gas in public. After a colostomy, there is no sphincter muscle to control emissions of gas, so noise and air can escape unexpectedly. When an ostomy renders you helpless to prevent this, you might think you can never leave the privacy of your home. This is not true. You are still in control of your digestive system, but there are new ways of exerting that control.

Having a colostomy appliance does not mean you will emit uncontrolled odors and noises. Noise can be muffled sometimes by pushing your hand against the stoma. Odors will not escape if you make sure the appliance fits well and that it is sealed around the stoma. Stoma caps have charcoal filter devices to serve as a deodorant for just this reason. Also, ask your physician about supplementing your diet with activated charcoal tablets. If you take two of these after meals, they can reduce the volume of gas by as much as 75 percent, and they deodorize any odors. Activated charcoal tablets work by absorbing gas and odors, but they might also absorb certain medications you are taking. This is why you need to check with your physician first.

Ask your doctor, ET nurse, or hospital dietitian for recommendations in menu planning that will reduce the amount of gas in your diet. You can also get information from the National Clearing House for Digestive Diseases (the address is in Appendix I). Some general recommendations include:

- Avoid gas-producing foods, such as broccoli, beans, cheese, and beer.
- Do not gulp your food. Take small bites and chew slowly.
- Get plenty of regular exercise, like walking.
- Eat foods that have a natural deodorant such as applesauce, cranberry juice, and yogurt.

This is one of the conditions you can discuss with other ostomates and is a good reason to belong to the colostomy club in your area. It can always help you to talk with people who have had the same kinds of fears and who will help you learn how to overcome them.

YOUR LOCAL COLOSTOMY CLUB

While not everybody with a colostomy has cancer, coping with lifestyle adjustments caused by colostomy has the same effect whether it was caused by cancer or ulcerative colitis. There is a very active and dynamic network of support across the country for people with ostomies. There are local chapters, publications, meetings, and a vast network for exchanging information.

Others with colostomies can share their experiences with you, tell you how they coped with their fear of being different and what kinds of clothing they wear to conceal the pouch. You can ask them how they coped with intimacy and sexuality and with work, recreational activity, and social life. One woman, a devout Catholic, said she was afraid to go to Mass at her church because her colon might make noise unexpectedly. A businessman expressed the same fear. How could he lead a business meeting with the fear of offending others? All of these problems have been experienced and overcome by other ostomates, so it is helpful to talk with them.

The United Ostomy Association can send a volunteer—who also had a colostomy—who matches your own age and background to help you through the initial period of adjustment. (The phone number and address are in Appendix 1.)

17

GOING BACK TO WORK

There are more than eight million cancer survivors in the United States, and the number grows daily as cancer treatment becomes more effective and cancer is increasingly cured because of early detection. More than 80 percent of them return to work after treatment. All occupations and professions include cancer survivors, yet many people still believe the myths that cancer is contagious, that you will not be able to work after you have had cancer, or that you will be taking sick days all too frequently. While there are more and more enlightened employers, there are some still in the dark ages.

Colorectal surgery can mean you will be out of work for a month or more. Radiation therapy can take seven weeks, and chemotherapy as much as a year. Nevertheless, you should expect to continue to work at your job. You might need to take one or two sick days or vacation days right after each chemotherapy treatment at the beginning of each treatment cycle, so once a month you might feel bad. But with proper scheduling, such as Friday afternoon treatments, you should be able to work right through. Remember, everybody is unique. You might feel no side effects at all from chemotherapy.

Radiation therapy must be taken every day, so this may be a more intense seven weeks. If you are going through radiation therapy, you might feel tired, but go to work anyway. Maybe you can schedule treatments for the end of the day and then go to bed earlier than normal when you get home. Many people, however, must have their treatment in the morning, and then they go to work with no problem. Just give yourself a break. You are not expected to be a dynamo every day. If you are drooping in the afternoon, take a short rest, even if it is just to sit somewhere quiet and shut your eyes for 10 minutes. If nausea is intense and medications do not help, then you might need to take a sick leave for the duration of the therapy.

If you have had a colostomy, you have one more adjustment to make, but there is no reason you cannot work and carry on your life just as you did before. Nobody has to know if you are an ostomate! You will not offend co-workers with unpleasant smells or bulges in your clothing. As mentioned earlier, there are more than a million ostomates from all walks of life who lead active, normal lives.

COMMUNICATING WITH YOUR CO-WORKERS

How you handle others depends on you and on them, as well as on the particular environment in which you work. If you are in a high-stress job like that of a Wall Street securities analyst, or if you are a trial attorney where your image has a lot to do with your performance, then you might not want to talk with any of your co-workers about your illness and treatment. If you work in the helping professions, it might be easier for you to share some of your feelings with people around you.

But if there are people with whom you can share confidences on the job, then let them know what you are going through. One of the best things to do is to tell your co-workers what is going on before your treatment and to keep in touch with them right after your surgery and during chemotherapy. Let them know that what you are doing is only temporary, like being treated for any other disease, that you are looking forward to coming back to work, and that you appreciate their concern. Educate them about your cancer and your treatment so they will understand what you are dealing with—and what you are not dealing with. If you must come in late or leave early or if you use your lunch hour for radiation treatments, say you are getting treatment, but you expect to be fine.

You might be in a large organization where there are already many other cancer survivors. In that case, you can seek out those others and perhaps even form a workplace support group. This can be a way to find mutual emotional support. And it might provide a forum for those co-workers who learn that they have cancer.

IF YOU ENCOUNTER DISCRIMINATION ON THE JOB

The six million cancer survivors who return to work are just as productive as other workers on any job, and they are not absent any more than usual. However, one in every four cancer survivors experiences some form of job discrimination. If this happens to you, there are laws to protect you and organizations that can help you.

In 1992, the Americans with Disabilities Act (ADA) went into effect. This law bans discrimination by employers against qualified workers who have disabilities or histories of disabilities. The law applies to private employers with 15 or more workers. Although cancer is not considered a disability, some employers obviously do, so it is covered by this law.

Federal employees have been covered since 1973, but private employers were not required to conform to these rules until 1992. The earlier law, the Federal Rehabilitation Act of 1973, also offers protection to employees of the federal government or companies that receive federal funds. This protects handicapped workers, including cancer survivors, in hiring policies, promotions, transfers, and layoffs.

The ADA was designed primarily to allow 14 million Americans with physical or mental handicaps to be gainfully employed, and there will be years of litigation before the inequities in the workplace are fixed. It is estimated that less than 14 percent of that population have been employed. Now, faced with a federal mandate, employers must hire—and not fire—people who are able to do their particular job. And, if disabilities are an obstacle, the employer must provide whatever practical adjustments are necessary, such as ramps, special furniture, or time to rest. Included in this mandate is flexible working hours, so if you are able to work during your treatment but you need time off to get that treatment, such as an hour or two for radiation therapy every day, then your employer must give you that time, even if he or she requests that you make up the extra hours at another time.

If you suspect your employer is encouraging you to retire early or to look for another job, or if he or she has used an unfair excuse to fire you, file a complaint with the Equal Employment Opportunities Commission (EEOC). In this age of downsizing, this kind of discrimination is often disguised, so enforcement is necessary. People are laid off if employers think they will need more benefits or they will often be out sick. One woman who had a colectomy shortly before she turned 65, was asked to retire at 65 even though she wanted to continue working. The end of work also meant the end of her benefits at this particular job; yet when she questioned the employer, she was told that a mandatory retirement ruling had just been established. This woman was deprived of her benefits as well as a job she had planned to enjoy for several more years. She also had a clear-cut case of discrimination to fight.

If you feel your job was terminated because of your illness, talk with the affirmative action officers where you work and let them know that you believe they you were unjustly laid off. They cannot retaliate by firing you. Look around the workplace for comparisons, too. Did they let another employee return after a heart attack? Did someone return to work after back surgery? If they do not reinstate you, file complaints with your state human rights commission within 180 days and with the EEOC within 300 days. Find a plaintiff's attorney to help you file this. Very often, an attorney will take on this kind of case without a fee and then get a percentage of the settlement later.

You can call the EEOC at 1-800-USA-EEOC (1-800-872-3362). And the National Cancer Institute's (NCI) guide *Facing Forward* has work-related information that might help you.

Your local American Cancer Society (ACS) chapter might be able to provide you with state-specific information pamphlets about federal and state law—including a copy of the recent ADA. Ask the ACS for their booklet explaining the ADA and your legal rights pertaining to jobs and health insurance. *Cancer: Your Job, Insurance, and the Law* is another helpful ACS publication.

The National Coalition for Cancer Survivorship (NCCS), at 1-301-585-2616, is an organization that offers information and sometimes legal referrals. Your hospital social workers might also know about laws in your state and the agencies involved in enforcing those laws. And also contact your congressional representative or senator for assistance.

WILL YOU BE ABLE TO CHANGE JOBS?

If you are looking for a new job, you do not have to reveal any information about your cancer treatment. In general, an employer cannot require preemployment physical examinations designed to screen out people with disabilities or medical histories of cancer. They can ask you medical questions only after you are offered employment and only if the questions relate specifically to the job. For example, they cannot ask you to reveal anything about your colon cancer or colostomy or chemotherapy if it is not relevant to, for example, your ability to work at your computer. You might have concerns yourself if you are a truck driver and are required to wear a seat belt across your abdomen for long periods of time, but you do not need to offer this information. It is up to you to decide if you can tolerate this condition. If you are turned down for a new job for reasons you believe are false, then you should protest. Do not discuss your health at a job interview.

In 1993, the EEOC declared that employers cannot refuse to hire people with disabilities and that people with disabilities must have equal access to health insurance. The EEOC also said they would enforce the 1992 ADA to curb discrimination by employers and insurers. (See Appendix III for more information about health insurance.)

There are lawyers who specialize as advocates and litigators on behalf of people with catastrophic illness. They can help you understand your rights under the ADA and under your state Human Rights Law and Family and Medical Leave Act—your rights to "reasonable accommodation" and what that means in the workplace, how to handle job interviews, and what to tell your employer—and what health benefits fall under the Employee Retirement Income Security Act (ERISA).

18

REVERSING SEXUAL SIDE EFFECTS OF TREATMENT

S ome colon cancer treatment can have a significant impact on a patient's sexuality when surgery and/or radiation interferes with the sacral nerves that are bundled at the base of the spine. These nerves, which are crucial to sexual functioning, are often severed when surgery must remove cancer from a low section of the colon or from the rectum.

In addition, radiation treatment to the pelvic area can damage blood vessels needed by men to achieve an erection. Radiation accelerates atherosclerosis and produces a reaction in the walls of the arteries that causes them to become calloused and thickened. The lumen (passageway) becomes obstructed, and in this condition the vessels are unable to transport blood in and out of the penis.

The effect of such damage to nerves and blood vessels in women is less drastic because they have no external organ that must function to assert sexual desire. The nerve damage in the pelvic area might reduce the actual physical sensation of sexual excitement. And a reduced blood flow to the labia, clitoris, and other parts of the genitals might inhibit arousal and lubrication. This can result in vaginal dryness and irritation, but women can counteract this condition by using a lubricant and by exploring other erogenous zones with their partners.

Men, on the other hand, might have to explore alternate methods of achieving an erection. Explanations of just how a penis becomes erect have been revised over time, but it is generally believed that the blood circulation changes when a man is aroused by physical or psychological means. More blood flows in and less flow out, and this makes the penis hard. This increased blood flow causes spaces in the penis filled with spongy tissue called *corporal bodies* to expand. The expansion compresses some veins, trapping blood in the penis and maintaining the firmness or the erection.

However, it is a complex dynamic involving nerves, blood vessels, and voluntary and involuntary reactions. The veins, arteries, and nerves must be intact and healthy to achieve and maintain an erection. Damage to these vessels inhibits the ability either to fill the penis with blood to achieve an erection or to trap the blood inside the penis in order to maintain the erection. Nerves and blood vessels in the sacral area also connect the impulses to the brain.

After radical surgery or radiation, most of these nerves and blood vessels become inoperable on their own, so they need some help. It is extremely important for men to talk with their surgeons or radiation oncologists in advance of treatment about what to expect and to seek out advice from their urologist so they will know how to cope with these side effects. This way they will know in advance that this is not a hopeless situation.

There are many options available for continuing a normal sex life with the help of external vacuum devices, penile prosthesis implants, or pharmacological self-injections. Urologists who specialize in sexual dysfunction are available in most major medical centers. There are also sex therapists who can help with the emotional adjustment to this new way of achieving erection. Numerous books and videos are available to educate patients about how to restore intimacy and sex to their lives by adapting to new methods. Some resources are listed at the end of this chapter.

VACUUM ERECTION DEVICE

A vacuum erection device (VED) is a simple mechanical device with a cylinder, a rubber band, and a pump. When the cylinder is fitted over the penis, air is pumped in and a vacuum is created. The vacuum draws blood into the penis, so an erection can be achieved. Then the penis is clamped off at the base with a band.

The results differ somewhat from a normal erection. For example, the penis may feel slightly cold, it might be larger in circumference, and it will pivot at the base. The penis is not stiff at the base but is very hard at the end. Veins might be distended, and it might look blue. Sometimes men notice a numbness while the constriction is in place, but this does not usually decrease pleasure. Additionally, ejaculate might not be able to flow until the constriction bands are removed.

This vacuum device provides only a hard penis. It will not affect sexual desire or allow a man to reach an orgasm if he is otherwise unable. However, the device does not prevent a man from reaching an orgasm, and some men find it easier to reach orgasm when they use the device. And a few find it more difficult. The device should not be considered a reliable contraceptive even though the constriction blocks the flow of semen in most men.

An advantage of vacuum therapy is that it mimics the natural process and allows complete control of when a man wants the erection and when he wants it to end. Some men—and their partners—believe it is better than nothing, while others say it seems mechanical and artificial. The major disadvantage, however, is that time is taken away from foreplay to use the pump, and some men feel that this ruins the mood.

PHARMACOLOGIC ERECTION PROGRAMS

Men who find the vacuum system less than desirable because it leaves them tumescent rather than firm might prefer a pharmacologic erection program (PAP). By injecting a drug—Caverject is the most common—into the side of the penis, an erection can be achieved and sustained.

The drugs are like the vasodilators used to treat heart conditions. They open up or dilate the blood vessels to allow blood to flow into the penis. Some drugs achieve this by relaxing the muscle cells in the arterial walls. This relaxation causes increased blood flow into the penis. At the same time, the blood that is carried out of the penis by the veins is reduced so that blood is trapped in the penis and the erection is maintained for a period that could range from 20 minutes to an hour and a half.

The penile injection can be administered before or after foreplay, and men are encouraged to experiment to see what works best. An erection occurs from 10 to 20 minutes after the injection, but some men might require a 30-minute wait before getting a fully rigid erection. The amount of time it takes generally correlates with the extent of arterial blockage.

The penile injection system requires training and surveillance by a physician. To begin generally requires two office visits designed to teach men how to give themselves the injection and to test their response to the drug. Finding the correct dosage is vitally important to the effectiveness of this system. Too little will not be effective, and too much could cause an erection to last too long and be possibly painful. During initial testing, the urologist might use the Doppler ultrasound test to scan the penis in its flaccid state and then again after an injection to measure the artery and note the difference in diameter. Then the physician will provide the patient with a prescription for disposable sterile syringes and needles.

It is important for men to visit their physician every three months to review their technique and for examination of the penis to be sure there are no side effects. Injections should not exceed 12 a month, and it is best if they are evenly spaced. The site should be alternated between the right side and left side of the penis to minimize scarring.

There are two types of potential side effects of the penile injection program. The first is simply that, whenever a needle is stuck in the body, a bruise can develop. Over time a small nodule or lump can develop at the site of repeated injection, and plaque might develop at the site. If the injection is not done properly, air can be injected into the veins; but this will cease eventually and cause no harm.

The second type of side effect results from the medication itself. The worst side effect is a prolonged erection. Some of the drugs used can produce a painful, sustained, prolonged erection, known as *priapism*. Priapism can last longer than four hours, and it requires immediate medical attention. This usually occurs early in the program when the patient and his physician are trying to find the right dose. Priapism is easy to reverse when treated early. But with proper education and testing in the doctor's office, the correct

168

amount of drug will be prescribed, and priapism should not be a problem.

Other side effects, which are very rare, include dizziness or headache or an increase in liver enzymes. Also extremely rare, is a slight, dull ache in the penis, but this usually subsides after about 15 minutes.

There is a high response rate (80 percent) to the penile injection system, but there is also a high dropout rate (30 to 50 percent) over the long term. Some men say it is unnatural, and they or their partners are afraid to touch their penis. Others claim they felt they were not in control.

Before you consider using the penile injection system, consider your own manual dexterity, your past medical history, and genital anatomy. This system *would not* be appropriate for you if:

- You have sickle cell disease.
- You have poor vision.
- You have poor manual dexterity.
- You are unwilling to follow instructions, which can create potential for misuse.

There are more than 40 centers all around the country that specialize in correcting sexual dysfunction with the penile injection system. Ask your urologist for information, and consult a book called *Making Love Again,* by J. Francois Eid, M.D., Director, Erectile Dysfunction Unit, The New York Hospital-Cornell Medical Center, 428 East 72nd Street, Suite 400, New York, NY 10021 (1-212-746-5473).

PENILE PROSTHESES

There are two types of penile prostheses that can be implanted surgically. Each is made of silicone, adapts well to the body, and has a very low risk of infection. One type leaves a man with a permanent erection. He can bend his penis to flatten it, but it will remain hard.

The other type, the two-cylinder prosthesis, can leave the penis erect or flaccid. One cylinder is implanted in the penis, and the other is implanted in the pelvic area. A hardening agent is transferred from one cylinder to the other when the prosthesis is activated. This is done by squeezing the head of the penis where the pump is located. Fluid is then released from the other cylinder to make the penis erect. To turn off the erection, the penis can simply be bent downward and the fluid will leave the penile cylinder and return to the storage cylinder.

Surgical implantation requires about three days in the hospital. Men feel pain or discomfort for several days until they get used to it and the surgery heals. The first erection can be painful, but it gets easier as men get used to it. The main advantage of such prostheses is that a man can have an erection for as long as he needs it.

SEX AFTER COLOSTOMY

A colostomy in no way interferes with normal sexual functioning, but often couples feel inhibited by the presence of the pouch. The pouch can usually be removed during that time or camouflaged in a variety of ways. Women can wear specially designed lingerie that conceals the pouch. Some men find that simply wearing a tee shirt is enough to cover their stoma or pouch and keep it out of mind. Medical supply houses that carry ostomy appliances usually also carry a line of intimate apparel designed to hide the pouch.

The most important element, of course, is the ability of you and your partner to be willing to experiment and to try new positions, and new forms of intimacy. Keep your stoma clean, and be sure your appliance fits properly so you do not spring a leak if you are leaned on. If that happens, just jump into the shower and start over.

The United Ostomy Association has two illustrated booklets that can help you: *Sex and the Female Ostomate* and *Sex and the Male Ostomate*. These booklets address concerns about sexual intimacy, potential solutions to problems, and resources for finding more help. The association also publishes brochures for gay and lesbian ostomates and for single ostomates. (See Appendix 1 for the address of the United Ostomy Association.)

GETTING OVER THE EMOTIONAL HURDLES

Studies have shown that in general, people who enjoyed a good sex life before cancer treatment will find a way to continue that enjoyment. There are many options, but it is vitally important for the patient and his or her partner to participate together in any discussions or therapy geared around sexuality. Affection and intimacy are important during recovery.

Impotence, even when it can be reversed, can create psychological problems to compound the situation. Men worry about their sexuality, but few are able to talk about this, and there is help for it. Even when men realize they need to get help—medical help—or lose their marriages, it is hard for them to talk. Women generally have the advantage of being better able to talk about any problems they might be having and in knowing how to seek help. It is important for men to communicate their concerns with their doctor as well as their partner.

COST OF TREATMENT

Some insurance coverage still does not recognize that sexual dysfunction is a medical condition. This is the result of years of thinking "it is all in your head"—an emotional problem rather than a medical one. The fact is that a very small percentage of impotence problems have psychological causes. One in 10 men are impotent as a result of health problems, such as high blood pressure, diabetes, spinal cord injuries, and even the side effects of certain medications. Now, most medical insurance plans cover the cost of treatment.

A vacuum device costs from $400 to $500, depending on whether it is the battery-assisted model or manual unit. It is covered by Medicare and most health insurance. Penile injections cost anywhere from $5 to $10 per injection, depending on the medication used. It could cost about $200 for a two-month supply of drugs and syringes, plus doctor visits. Penile implants, requiring surgery, are naturally more costly.

FINDING INFORMATION AND TREATMENT

There are many specialists who treat sexual dysfunction in men and women. For men, a visit to their urologist would be a first step. The urologist would then refer the patient to a subspecialist.

Women would visit their gynecologist to check the condition of their genital area, and to find out if anything can be done physically to improve their enjoyment of sex.

There are sex therapists who can counsel about the emotional aspects of sexual dysfunction, but it is important to check their credentials first. The following list is a good place to start in your search for information.

The American Association of Sex Educators, Counselors, and Therapists (AASECT)

11 Dupont Circle, NW
Suite 220
Washington, DC 20036
1-202-462-1171

It offers assistance in finding a sex therapist.

The Impotence Information Center

PO Box 9
Dept. USA
Minneapolis, MN 55440
1-800-843-4315

They can help you find a support group in your area.

Impotence Anonymous

119 S. Ruth St.
Maryville, TN 37801-5746

This group has chapters throughout the United States. Send a stamped self-addressed envelop for list of chapters.

Potency Restored

c/o Giulio Scarzella, M.D.
8630 Fenton Street, Suite 218
Silver Spring, MD 10910

Write for information about chapters in many states.

Recovery of Male Potency (ROMP)

c/o Grace Hospital
18700 Meyers Rd.
Detroit, MI 48235
1-800-TEL-ROMP outside Michigan
1-313-927-3219 for Michigan residents

They have chapters in many states.

Not for Men Only

c/o Mercy Hospital and Medical Center
Stevenson Expressway at King Drive
Chicago, IL 60616
1-800-448-8664 outside Chicago
1-312-567-5567 for Illinois residents

Groups for couples as well as groups for men or women.

The American Cancer Society has two excellent booklets about sexuality after cancer treatment. Call your local branch to get a copy.

Sexuality and Cancer: For the Woman Who Has Cancer and Her Partner

Sexuality and Cancer: For the Man Who Has Cancer and His Partner

19

PROTECTING YOUR FAMILY FROM COLON CANCER

It is estimated that up to 10 percent of all cancers result from an inherited gene change, and this might be higher for colon cancer. Everyone is at risk for cancer (1 in 3 in a lifetime), but some people have the added risk of an inherited predisposition to genetic mutations.

Until colon cancer can be identified with a simple test, enhanced surveillance of high-risk individuals should make it possible to identify a cancer at its earliest, and curable, stage. It is expected that within a few years, a simple blood test will be sufficient to determine whether a child has inherited susceptibility for the disease.

The gene that causes the predisposition can be inherited, but that alone is not enough to produce a cancer. A cell becomes malignant only after multiple gene changes have occurred.

SPORADIC COLON CANCER IN FAMILIES

In populations with high incidence of colon cancer, familial factors seem to play a strong role, and that role might be affected by the environment. In Israel, for example, European-born Jews have a higher incidence of colon cancer than non-European-born Jews. But genetic factors seem to have more impact in the latter group.

If a person has one first-degree relative—sibling, parent, or child—with colon cancer, the odds of that person getting cancer are high, almost twice as high as the rest of the population, and screening for prevention is the only cure. With two affected first-degree relatives, the incidence of adenomas is more than five times higher. An Australian case control study found that the odds ratio for colon cancer was 1.8 for one affected first-degree relative and 5.7 for two.

A large number of individuals, their spouses, and first-degree relatives were screened with flexible sigmoidoscopy, and a family history had significant impact. This study implied that 19 percent of the population is more susceptible to colonic neoplasia on a familial basis.

It is important to tell your relatives (especially your children and siblings) that you have colon cancer and to encourage them to get regular screenings. Share your colon cancer history with them, and encourage them to share it with their own doctors so that they will be diligent about getting digital rectal exams, fecal occult blood tests (FOBT), and regular sigmoidoscopies. This is not only for families with the inherited familial polyposis, which accounts for only 1 percent of colon cancer patients, because studies have shown that anyone with a first- or second-degree relative with colon cancer is at greater risk.

Recent research has identified several of the genes predisposing to particular cancers—breast cancer, for example. Testing to detect carriers of those mutations will be possible in the near future. What this will mean is that a family with cancer can be defined in terms of its predisposition mutation. Then it will be possible to determine which family members have, or have not, inherited that mutation.

FAMILIAL ADENOMATOUS POLYPOSIS OR GARDNER'S SYNDROME

Occasionally patients will have a familial (inherited) adenomatous polyposis (FAP) syndrome. In these conditions, multiple colonic and rectal polyps are present. Polyps might involve the stomach and small intestine as well, and there is often a family history of colonic and rectal polyps and possibly of colon cancer. These syndromes can differ widely in their clinical manifestations, patterns of inheritance, types and locations of polyps, and predisposition, if any, to the development of carcinoma of the colon, rectum, and other parts of the gastrointestinal tract.

FAP is characterized by the development of multiple small polyps—as many as hundreds of thousands—from the mucous membrane of the colon and rectum. In time, one or more of these polyps will become cancer, so they must be removed. It is now standard practice to examine all children born to a FAP patient.

Your family members—including children over age 10—should follow up with colonoscopy every two years until they are 40, then three to five years until age 60. Adenomatous polyps develop when a child is between 10 and 20. If they have not appeared by age 40, the changes of getting colon cancer from FAP are greatly reduced.

Only children born to you need to be examined because the disease does not skip generations. Your grandchildren are not at risk unless one of their parents had the disease. If one parent carries the gene for FAP—chromosome number 5—each child has a 50/50 chance of getting it. However, this risk drops with age to only 10 percent if no polyps are found in the rectum by age 18. And if they do not appear by age 30, the risk drops to 3 percent.

FAP and Gardner's syndrome are related conditions that likely stem from the same genetic syndrome. They are inherited in an autosomal (not sex-linked) dominant pattern with affected individuals developing hundreds of colon and rectal polyps in the first three decades of life. Polyps often commonly occur in the stomach and small intestine as well. Unless the colon and rectum are surgically removed, all of these patients will eventually develop colon and rectal cancer.

Patients with Gardner's syndrome are also more likely to have adenomatous polyps in the proximal small intestine, especially in the area where the bile duct and pancreatic duct drain into the duodenum. Surveillance colonoscopy is usually begun in childhood around the age of 10 in family members believed to have this disorder. Total proctocolectomy with an anal sphincter-sparing operation is indicated for these patients by the time they reach their twenties. (See Chapter 8 about this prophylactic surgery.)

OTHER SYNDROMES

Turcot syndrome is a rare disorder in which colonic and rectal polyposis is associated with brain tumors. The stomach and small intestine are usually not involved. Cancer predisposition exists. The disorder might be inherited in a recessive or dominant pattern. Surveillance and treatment recommendations are similar to those of FAP.

Peutz-Jeghers syndrome involves polyps primarily in the small intestine with some spillover into the stomach and colon. Patients with this syndrome can be identified by pigmented plaques—like dark freckles—of their gums and lips. They also might have bladder and nasal polyps. Surgery may be necessary because of the development of intestinal obstruction and bleeding from the small intestinal polyps. As the cancer predisposition is low—less than a 3 percent risk—prophylactic surgery is not usually recommended.

Other polyposis syndromes exist, but these have little or no increased risk of colon and rectal cancer. These include juvenile polyposis; von Recklinghausen's disease, in which neurofibromas involve the stomach, small bowel, and skin; and Cronkhite-Canada syndrome, in which inflammatory polyps of the small bowel, stomach, and colon might be associated with baldness, excessive skin pigmentation, and fingernail changes. Because of the rarity of all polyposis syndromes, expert medical attention, usually available at a university medical center, is desirable for proper diagnosis and treatment guidelines.

Hereditary nonpolyposis colorectal cancer (HNPCC), or Lynch syndrome, is a cancer syndrome in which nearly all affected members develop cancer, but in different ways than FAP families. Lynch syndrome families develop multiple primary polyps, both synchronous and metachronous, mostly in the proximal colon, that is, the portion closer to the cecum. There are two types: Lynch syndrome I is an early-onset cancer of the colon, and Lynch syndrome II is characterized by early-onset cancer at other sites, including the endometrium (uterus lining), ovaries, upper urinary tract, small intestine, and stomach. The presence of these tumors tends to cluster in certain families, underscoring the need to obtain detailed information on tumor development.

177

Teenaged patients occasionally develop malignant tumors before Lynch syndrome develops in their parents. Because it is sometimes assumed a generation was skipped, this can confuse diagnosis. With Lynch syndrome, the history of the entire family, including grandparents, aunts and uncles, and children, must be understood.

While the majority of colon cancers in the general population occur in the sigmoid area, in Lynch syndrome patients, 65 percent to 88 percent of the tumors occur in the cecum colon.

COLON CANCER REGISTRIES

Colon cancer registries contain the names of hundreds of people, and their families, who have had colon and rectal cancer. These registries primarily exist for research tools for scientists studying the genetics of colon cancer. It allows them to make an analysis of a family tree (or pedigree) of colon cancer patients. This sometimes makes it possible to determine a mathematical risk of cancer for any individual in that family. With multiple family members available to the registry researchers, simple blood tests make it possible to directly analyze the genetic material (DNA)—a first step in defining which cancer predisposition gene might be inherited in a particular family.

If you want to sign up and join a registry with the notion that it might advance the cause of colon cancer research, ask your treatment team which one is appropriate for you.

THE FUTURE FOR YOU AND YOUR FAMILY

Urge your family to be screened because they are at risk, and tell your friends to be aware of how to prevent a disease that does not have to take so many lives, even though 5 to 6 percent of the population will get it.

It is hoped that just as Medicare finally (in 1992) began covering the cost of annual screening mammograms for breast cancer, this same type of screening for early detection of colon cancer can save lives.

To provide FOBT and flexible sigmoidoscopy to approximately 60 million Americans over 50 would cost about three billion dollars a year in a national prevention program. But, ironically, that is less than the nearly four billion dollars on direct costs of colon cancer treatment (1990).

Every day, medical science learns more about treating cancer. We hope that, in our lifetime, we will no longer have to treat it—that it can truly be prevented. We hope you find this book helpful, and we hope you take our advice to get the best treatment you can and take good care of yourself.

It is hoped that, as treatment improves, as doctors learn how to educate their patients as well as care for them, as patients take more responsibility for their care, as preventive health care becomes more widespread, and as health insurance becomes more accessible and affordable, colon cancer can be eliminated.

In the meantime, carry the message with you wherever you go. **Early detection is the cure.**

INFORMATION RESOURCES ABOUT COLON CANCER

A wide network of information resources about colon cancer is available. People who answer telephone hotlines are specially trained to provide up-to-date information and most of these agencies can provide the information in Spanish as well as English (Occasionally in other languages). If you call with a question or need a referral, they can help you. If they cannot help, they will know who can.

NCI Cancer Information Service Hotline—1-800-4-CANCER (1-800-422-6237)

The National Cancer Institute (NCI) is the primary federal agency for cancer research and information on everything from clinical trials to new drugs. The hotline is operated by a network of authorized comprehensive cancer centers and will connect you with the one nearest you. The NCI keeps an up-to-date file of available resources and physicians working with all types of cancer. The hotline operates weekdays only, from 9 A.M. to 4:30 P.M., Eastern standard time.

Information is from PDQ, a computer service that gives up-to-date information on cancer treatment. PDQ is a service for cancer patients and their families and for doctors, nurses, and other healthcare professionals. PDQ information is reviewed each month by cancer experts and is updated when the information changes. PDQ also lists information about research on new treatments (clinical trials), doctors who treat cancer, and hospitals with cancer programs.

You can also obtain information from the NCI by fax or through the Internet:

CancerFax (1-301-402-5874) is a way to obtain PDQ information statements in English or Spanish using a fax machine. It contains fact sheets on various cancer topics from the NCI's office of cancer communications. CancerFax operates 24 hours a day, seven days a week, with no charge other than the telephone call. For a fact sheet explaining how to use CancerFax, call 1-800-4-CANCER.

CancerNet can be accessed at cancernet@icicc.nci.nih.gov — enter the word HELP in the BODY of the E-mail message (or Spanish to receive the information in Spanish). CancerNet will send you a return E-mail message containing the contents list of materials available through CancerNet. There is no charge.

American Cancer Society—1-800-ACS-2345 (1-800-227-2345) for your local chapter

With 3,400 chapters in the United States, this is the largest voluntary health agency in the world. ACS sponsors research, education, and patient-service programs, including transportation to and from treatment, support groups, and equipment loans. It is usually a good way to find out what resources are available in your community. They have affiliated programs:

Look Good, Feel Better—**1-800-395-LOOK (1-800-395-5665) or your local ACS chapter**—is a hotline for women undergoing chemotherapy, operated weekdays from 9 A.M. and 5 P.M. Eastern standard time. They offer referrals to free workshops in 50 states that provide practical advice from hair and makeup professionals. Information is available in English and Spanish. They can identify certain salons in your area where a specialist will be sent to assist you with your hair and makeup.

I Can Cope is a patient- and family-education program with series of classes, often held at a local hospital. Information is provided by physicians, nurses, social workers, and community representatives. The focus is education about your diagnosis and treatment and assistance with coping with cancer as a physical and emotional challenge.

Cancer Care national toll-free counseling line—1-800-813-HOPE (1-800-813-4673)

1180 Avenue of the Americas
New York, NY 10036
1-212-221-3300

Cancer Care is a voluntary agency, founded in 1944, dedicated to providing support for cancer patients and their families and friends, as well as education for the general public. It offers professional social work counseling and guidance free of charge and serves about 50,000 people a year. Cancer Care focuses on helping cancer patients—at any stage of illness—cope with the emotional, social, and financial burdens of cancer.

Financial assistance of nearly $1.4 million is provided annually to eligible families to help with home care, transportation, pain medication, and medical treatment costs.

A nationwide counseling line—offered in English, Spanish, and Yiddish—provides emotional support; problem solving; guidance with doctor-patient communication, second opinions, and finding your way through the healthcare system; information and referral to local community resources; computerized resource directory; and practical guidelines for obtaining home care, transportation to treatment, and access to entitlements.

Programs of professional consultation and education, community education and awareness, social research, and public policy are conducted on a local and national level. Cancer Care also provides free education materials on a range of cancer diagnoses and treatment options and telephone support groups and educational seminars for patients, family members, and caregivers.

Patient Advocates for Advanced Cancer Treatments (PAACT)
1143 Parmelee, NW
Grand Rapids, MI 49504
1-616-453-1477
Call for information.

National Coalition for Cancer Survivorship (NCCS)
1010 Wayne Avenue
Suite 300
Silver Spring, MD 20910
1-301-585-2616

This is a network of independent groups and individuals concerned with survivorship and support of cancer survivors and their loved ones. NCCS's primary goal is to promote a national awareness of issues affecting cancer survivors. Its objectives are to: Serve as a clearing house for information on services and materials for survivors, Advocate the rights and interests of cancer survivors, Encourage the study of survivorship, and Promote the development of cancer support activities.

American College of Surgeons Committee on Cancer
55 East Erie St.
Chicago, IL 60611

Write for a booklet listing approved cancer programs. Revised quarterly.

American Society of Colon and Rectal Surgeons
85 West Algonquin Road
Suite 550
Arlington Heights, IL 60005
1-847-290-9184

Call for brochure about surgery and list of certified surgeons in your area.

The Chemotherapy Foundation
183 Madison Avenue
New York, NY 10016
1-212-213-9292

Ask for their free 40-page booklet on chemotherapy. It explains in detail how chemotherapy works, what drugs are used, and more.

United Ostomy Association, Inc.
36 Executive Park
Suite 120
Irvine, CA 92714-6744
1-800-826-0826
1-714-660-8624
Fax 1-714-660-9262

The toll-free phone number operates from 7 A.M. to 4 P.M. Pacific standard time and offers basic information and referrals to local chapters. This national organization offers educational and psychological support for people with colostomies. It also provides advocacy and family support. Trained and certified home visitors can come to you before and/or after surgery. They will also help train your partner or spouse. More than 540 chapters throughout the United States and Canada provide newsletters, support groups, and visiting services.

Publishes *Ostomy Quarterly*, with news and information on ostomy management, human interest, nutrition tips, and new products.

National Digestive Diseases Clearinghouse
Box NDDIC
9000 Rockville Pike
Bethesda, MD 20892
1-301-654-3810

A branch of the National Institutes of Health, the National Digestive Diseases Clearinghouse answers questions and provides information through a wide variety of publications, for example, Document 50 suggests diet for colostomy patients trying to omit gas-forming foods from their meals. They also have booklets on colon cancer prevention and screening; high-fiber, low-fat diet; and living with colostomy.

The organization works with other patient organizations. Call for a list of their publications.

SOURCES OF FINANCIAL AID FOR COLON CANCER SCREENING AND TREATMENT

Where to Get Free or Low-Cost Screening

Many communities have hospitals or private foundations that periodically provide free or low-cost early detection opportunities such as fecal occult blood test (FOBT) or sigmoidoscopy. Check with your employer's health office, the social service department of your hospital, or your local American Cancer Society (ACS) to find out what is available in your area.

Financial Aid for Chemotherapy

Drug companies often provide chemotherapy drugs at low or no cost to people who cannot afford to pay for them. Your chemotherapist or your local ACS chapter might know about this. Your oncologist can also write for the Directory of Prescription Drug Indigent Programs, which can help locate drugs at low or no cost. This is published by the Pharmaceutical Manufacturer's Association in Washington, D.C.

Transportation to and from Treatments

Ask your local ACS chapter or your treatment team about transportation resources. In some communities, the ACS has a program called "Road to Recovery," designed for this purpose. Trained volunteer drivers take you to treatment and pick you up. There is also a national Corporate Angels program that provides long-distance air transportation to a treatment facility.

See Appendix 1 for information on Cancer Care, which provides financial aid to some cancer patients.

Other Sources of Aid

Help for a specific financial problem is usually available somewhere, but it will take some persistent digging and phone calling. Perhaps a family member can help. In addition to the cancer care agencies listed here, other potential sources are community service groups and fraternal and religious organizations in your own neighborhood, public welfare agencies, and state and federally funded medical programs, such as Medicaid and Medicare.

IF YOU HAVE MANAGED-CARE INSURANCE COVERAGE

The majority of the medically insured population is now enrolled in a managed-care insurance program, mostly through their place of employment. It is important that you understand how these health maintenance organizations (HMOs) affect your treatment options.

Test and Treatment Restrictions

HMOs generally require you to be treated only through referrals from your primary care physician. This can put a limitation on your choices of specialists and treatment options for colon cancer. You might be restricted only to the physicians listed in your HMO directory. This means you cannot visit an oncologist or surgeon unless that physician is in the same plan and is referred by the primary care physician. Sometimes HMO restrictions also mean you can seek treatment only in your own neighborhood, city, or state. You might prefer to go to another state where there is a state-of-the-art treatment center.

Another risk is the so-called "gag rule" that some managed-care plans require of physicians in their network. Some do not allow their physicians to tell patients about other possible treatment options. Because some of these restrictions have proven to be detrimental to good health care, states have begun passing laws to prevent HMOs from making such decisions. The rules are changing every day, and it is vital to your well-being to keep abreast of the changes in your medical insurance plan.

Here is an example of what you must be careful with if you are covered by an HMO plan. Suppose you have an endoscopic examination in the gastroenterology suite at a medical center. A polyp is removed and sent for biopsy, but the hospital's pathology fee is not covered by your insurer, which will only pay for pathology done by a particular outside commercial laboratory. However, if you are being treated in a comprehensive cancer center, your surgeon will not want to make a surgical decision based on a commercial laboratory biopsy. He or she will want one done in the same place where the screening was done. Physicians generally consider such outside commercial laboratories acceptable for analysis of potassium levels and other minor tests, but many doctors will not trust them for anything as critical as an accurate biopsy.

Doctors are used to working with other doctors whom they know as part of a multidisciplinary team to deal with a patient's problems. Mutual trust, a common hospital, complementary training, and professional competence are a part of the glue holding together these teams. Current trends in health insurance do not necessarily recognize these groups, and the teams could be fragmented if one or more physicians necessary to your care are not in your plan. This sometimes results in excess strain on the doctor-patient relationship if access to what is perceived as necessary or desirable by healthcare providers is limited by health insurance coverage. For example, if your surgeon must get the biopsy slides from another laboratory or hospital and then have them analyzed again, you will have to pay the cost of the second biopsy—your insurance will not cover it.

Always be sure to find out ahead of time what complications you will run into. You want to know that you are getting the best possible treatment—indeed the proper treatment.

Here is a hypothetical case: Suppose you had Duke's Stage B colon cancer, and the disease is removed by a surgical excision. Although the pathologist found no cancer outside the colon wall, the cancer did exist at the margin of resection. Nevertheless, you and your physicians discuss this situation. As mentioned in Chapter 11 (the chapter on chemotherapy), this is an area of medical controversy. Some physicians would prescribe adjuvant chemotherapy to be sure there are no cancer cells on their way to other organs. Others might say that the risk is so small it is not worth putting a patient through the months of chemotherapy. Ultimately, you and your physicians must make this decision.

However, you might be faced with rules made by your insurance company. It is quite possible that a particular HMO would not cover the cost of chemotherapy treatment for Duke's Stage B colon cancer. This same situation could arise if you and your physicians decide that a colon resection, requiring open abdominal surgery, would be a wise treatment decision in your case, but your insurance company rules say that you can only get a surgical resection if you have a more advanced stage of disease.

Many states have enacted laws to prevent managed care organizations from denying certain kinds of coverage to patients and from making decisions that should be made by doctors and patients. Here are some of the managed-care policies that have been reversed in some states as of the middle of 1996:

- A dozen states now guarantee a patient's right to go directly to certain types of specialists without first getting approval from a primary care physician, whom insurers consider a "gatekeeper." This prior approval severely limited patients' options in choosing the best and most appropriate care. The new legislation requires healthcare networks to accept any physician—any willing provider—who has appropriate credentials and agrees to abide by contract terms and conditions. This means that, if you have a doctor who is not in your plan but who is qualified to treat you, the insurance company must pay for the treatment.
- A number of states now require managed-care companies and their doctors to tell patients about financial incentives and rules that might affect their care.
- At least six states have outlawed the gag rules under which some HMOs threaten to dismiss doctors if they inform patients about alternative care that might add to the costs of treatment. Healthcare or insurance networks cannot restrict what information practitioners can give patients about care choices.

Before you begin treatment, call your HMO, and talk with the patient services department of your medical center. They can often help you get through the red tape and find out exactly what is covered and not covered.

Other Insurance Limitations

Medical insurance coverage varies, and even if you are fully covered, you might still have to pay a percentage of the costs for your care. A small copayment percentage on tens of thousands of dollars can leave you bankrupt. There could also be a limit to your coverage, and after the costs reach that limit, you are responsible for the rest of the payment.

Be sure you get all the coverage and benefits your policy provides. It is a good idea to read your policy and be familiar with it. Keep very careful records of all of your expenses. File claims immediately for covered costs. Many people do not do this and find later that they are confused about what they have claimed and not claimed. It is always more difficult to do this months later, because in our insurance system, the paperwork can become overwhelming.

If you need help in filing claims and understanding how to report your expenses, ask for help. There might be somebody in your family, a hospital worker, or a business associate who is up on how health insurance works.

Also, if any claim is turned down, file it again. Call the insurer and be sure to ask for an explanation of why you were turned down. This can happen because of an error in the filing of information from your doctor's office or the hospital or at the insurance company itself. Claims go through many hands. Always confirm conversations with insurance representatives in writing, or make detailed notes for your file after a telephone conversation.

Most treatment centers and hospitals have three sets of figures for each patient procedure: (1) what they charge the patient; (2) what the treatment costs them to provide; and (3) what they will receive from medical insurance companies. For this reason, there is some flexibility and you can probably negotiate a fair price in advance if you know you are going to have to come up with an enormous sum of money. So the advice here is to find out what all the charges are, how much your insurance will cover, and what remains for you to pay—and how to pay it. Will you be able to get help from an outside agency? Will the hospital let you pay in installments? Most are willing to arrange a convenient payment plan.

Getting Health Insurance after Colon Cancer

If you are turned down for health insurance coverage because you have had colon cancer, call your state department of insurance. It might be illegal in your state for an insurance carrier to reject you as long as you are able to pay the premiums. Laws are changing daily as health insurance undergoes changes. Many states are forcing insurers to accept anybody who applies and pays for health insurance, regardless of medical conditions for which they have been treated in the past. There are also companies that insure people with high medical expenses. These are often the Blue Cross, Blue Shield companies in each state. If you are turned down by any company, find out if they have an appeals process.

Before you leave any job that includes insurance coverage, be sure that you are covered by the new job or that you will be able to pick up insurance on your own. You will be covered by your last employer's insurance for 18 months, providing you pay the monthly premiums. This is covered by federal law, known as COBRA, the Consolidated Omnibus Budget Reconciliation Act.

If a new employer's insurance, or individual insurance of your own, will not cover you for a preexisting condition for a year, then keep the COBRA coverage and pay the premiums yourself, until your new policy kicks in. You must be able to pay for your follow-up care and surveillance, which can take several years and cost tens of thousands of dollars.

For a cancer survivor, health insurance must include, at the very least, these expenses:

- Inpatient hospital care, physician services, laboratory and X-ray services, inpatient psychiatric care, outpatient services, and nursing home care. Prescription drug coverage could be important if you will be taking a medication for a long period of time.

- The insurer should pay at least 80 percent of the covered services, except possibly for inpatient psychiatric care, which might require that you pay more than 20 percent. Also, the insurer should pay at least $250,000 for catastrophic illness coverage, with you paying no more than 30 percent of your income toward these expenses. Check on the limit, too. Some policies cover you up to a million dollars in a lifetime, and some have no lifetime cap.

There are many options for health insurance. If you are not covered by your employer or if you cannot afford individual coverage, look into fraternal and professional societies and organizations that often provide group coverage and lower rates. Try an independent insurance broker, or inquire about a high-risk pool.

Call your local Social Security office to find out costs covered by these federal insurance programs: Medicaid and Medicare. If you are over 65 or permanently disabled, you might qualify for Medicare, so call your local Social Security office or your city's office of the aging. If you are unemployed or in a low-income bracket, you might be eligible for Medicaid, but coverage differs from state to state. If you are a military veteran, inquire at the U.S. Department of Veterans Affairs.

To file insurance complaints if you think you have been treated unfairly, call your state department of insurance, or for managed care providers, call your state department of corporations, division of healthcare service plans.

APPENDIX 4

YOUR MEDICAL RECORDS AND THE LAW

Always have copies of your medical records. Your records are your files, and you will want to have them—or at least know what is in them—if you visit other doctors or hospitals. The most useful are your colonoscopy, pathology, and operative reports. You might want them with you, so that years later you will have easy access to them if you need them. You might want your family or other significant people to have access to your medical information in an emergency.

Federal law guarantees your right to your medical records. And this law is mandated by most states, as well, in spite of opposition of many doctors who claim patients would not understand the meaning of entries in their records. Your right of privacy is also protected, so that others cannot have your medical records without your knowledge and approval. Most hospitals have a medical records department, and they sometimes move slowly because a great deal of paper is handled here. If you want a copy of any or all of your medical records, you have to put the request in writing and complete a form supplied by the hospital. This legally protects both you and the hospital. You should be able to get copies of your records within a few days, however, and sooner if it is urgent. You are entitled to hospital records, doctor records, diagnostic records, X-ray films, pathology slides, all of it.

The best thing to do, as has been mentioned throughout this book, is to always get copies of your medical records after each procedure you have and as you progress through treatment.

Some doctors have no problem giving you copies. Others tell you to write them a letter requesting copies. They might charge a small processing fee. This is just their way of putting another barrier in the way. It is all a matter of style because you are entitled to your records. Just keep on insisting.

SOME HELPFUL BOOKS AND VIDEOS

Books

The PDR Family Guide to Nutrition and Health
Published in 1995 by the publishers of The Physicians' Desk Reference (PDR), this is an excellent guide with expert advice on fat, salt, and cholesterol. The book includes the latest research on cancer, the medical facts on healing with diet, and vital tips on energy, fitness, and weight loss and gain. This book is indispensable for anyone who wishes to maximize the beneficial impact of nutrition on health.

Facing Forward: A Guide for Cancer Survivors, NIH Publication No. 93-2424
This free 43-page booklet from the National Institutes of Health, National Cancer Institute (NCI) (revised October 1992) contains good solid information on continuing your health care after cancer, managing insurance issues, taking care of your feelings, earning a living, and moving ahead. You might find this in your hospital library, or you can write to the NCI at 9000 Rockville Pike, Bethesda, MD 20892.

Other publications from the NCI are:

Chemotherapy and You
Radiation Therapy and You
What Are Clinical Trials All About?
Eating Hints for Cancer Patients
Taking Time: Support for People with Cancer and the People Who Care about Them

When Cancer Recurs: Meeting the Challenge Again
Advanced Cancer: Living Each Day

Coping with an Ostomy: A Guide for Living
by Robert H. Phillips, Ph.D., Avery Publishing Group, Wayne, NJ.

Making Love Again
By J. Francois Eid, M.D., Director of the Erectile Dysfunction Unit at the New York Hospital-Cornell Medical Center in New York. (Brunner/Mazel, 1993)

Sexuality and Cancer: For the Woman Who Has Cancer and Her Partner
Sexuality and Cancer: For the Man Who Has Cancer and His Partner

Helpful books from the American Cancer Society.

Video

Colon and Rectal Cancer, video
Time Life Medical Personal Videos with Workbooks. These videos are widely available at supermarkets and drug stores for about $20.

Many medical centers have videos and books available to give to patients as part of their patient-education efforts; ask nurses and social workers about these. And many books and videos are also available from the organizations listed in Appendix 1.

Colon Cancer in Cyberspace

If you have a computer connected to the Internet, you will find many citations on colon cancer through Yahoo and Altavista search services. There are articles by medical professionals, as well as information and commentary from people who have the disease.

GLOSSARY OF COLON CANCER MEDICAL SPECIALISTS

Here is a list of definitions of medical specialties needed in the treatment of colon and rectal cancer.

Colorectal surgeon: A surgeon with additional training in the surgical treatment of diseases of the colon and rectum.

Endoscopist: A physician, usually a gastroenterologist, but occasionally a (colorectal) surgeon who performs endoscopy.

Gastroenterologist: An internist with two to three years of additional training in digestive diseases, including training in endoscopy.

General surgeon: A surgeon with training in all types of surgery, including that of the colon and rectum.

Medical oncologist: An internist with two to three years of additional training in the treatment of cancer, usually by chemotherapy.

Oncologic surgeon: A surgeon with additional training in the surgery of malignant neoplasms of all body systems.

Pathologist: A physician with training and expertise in interpreting biopsies and specimens removed from the body for the purpose of making a diagnosis.

Radiation oncologist (Radiation therapist): A physician with training and expertise in radiation therapy of malignancies.

Radiologist: A physician with training and expertise in performing and interpreting X rays.

GLOSSARY OF TERMS

adenoma: A polyp growing from glandular tissue in the mucous membrane of the colon.

adenopathy: Enlarged lymph nodes that might suggest presence of colon cancer. Also lymphadenopathy.

adjuvant therapy: Treatment given in addition to the primary therapy.

alopecia: Hair loss.

anastomosis: Surgical union of any two portions of the colon or rectum after the cancerous portion has been surgically removed.

aneuploid: Cell population that contains other than the normal amount of DNA material.

anterior resection: Resection of the rectosigmoid colon with low abdominal incision.

ascending colon: Portion of the colon after the cecum; located in the upper right side of the abdomen; leads into the transverse colon, which lies across the abdomen.

atypical hyperplasia: Excessive growth of cells; premalignant condition.

barium enema X ray: Procedure in which the colon is filled with an opaque fluid (barium) so that an X ray can be taken to see what is in the colon.

benign: A noncancerous condition.

biofeedback: Method of self-monitoring and controlling some bodily systems; used to reduce muscle tension, blood pressure, nausea, stress, and pain.

biopsy: Removal of tissue for histologic analysis, microscopic study, or pathologic evaluation.

bowel: Another name for the *intestine,* both large and small.

CA-15-3: Blood test used to find recurrence or metastasis; more suggestive of bone metastasis.

carcinoembryonic antigen (CEA): Substance that is sometimes found in increased amount in the blood of colorectal cancer patients.

carcinoma: Cancer that begins in the lining or covering tissues of an organ (epithelium) such as the colon.

CAT scan (CT scan): *Computerized axial tomography.* A cross-sectional X ray used in diagnosis and radiation treatment planning.

CEA assay: Blood test used to measure the level of carcinoembryonic antigen in the blood of colorectal cancer patients.

cecum: Beginning—or proximal portion—of the colon; located on the lower right side of the abdomen, where the small intestine empties into it.

chemotherapy: Systemic treatment with medications that reach every cell in the body.

chronic ulcerative colitis (CUC): Disease of all or part of the colon; can often be a risk factor for colon cancer.

Crohn's disease: Disease of the colon; can often be a risk factor for colon cancer.

clinical trials: Controlled research studies of cancer treatments on a fixed number of volunteer patients; designed to answer certain questions and to determine better ways to prevent, detect, or treat cancer.

colectomy: Surgery to remove all or part of the colon. In a *partial colectomy*, the surgeon removes only the cancerous part of the colon and a small mount—called a *margin*—of surrounding healthy tissue. See also *margins of resection*.

colonic irrigation: Flushing out the colon by inserting water into the colon via the anus.

colonoscope: A tube inserted through the anus and into the colon; used to diagnose diseases of the large intestine.

colonoscopy: Endoscopic visualization of the entire colon with a flexible, lighted instrument called a colonoscope.

colostomy: An opening created by a surgeon into the colon from the outside of the body; provides a new path for waste material to leave the body after part of the colon has been removed.

CTX: Medical shorthand for *chemotherapy treatment*.

cytology: Study of cells under the microscope.

cytotoxic: Type of substance toxic to cells; refers to drugs used in chemotherapy to kill or slow down the reproduction of cancer cells.

descending colon: Portion of the colon after the transverse colon and before the sigmoid and rectum; located in the upper left side of the abdomen.

differentiated: Resemblance of cancer cells to normal cells. Well-differentiated tumor cells closely resemble normal cells and are, therefore, believed to be less aggressive.

diffuse: Condition of cancer cells, as opposed to concentrated or organized. Cancer cells are spread out, thinly scattered over a large area.

digital rectal exam (DRE): Used to detect rectal cancer. The doctor inserts a lubricated, gloved finger into the rectum and feels for abnormal areas.

diploid: Cell population that contains the normal amount—1.00— of DNA material.

distal: Term that indicates direction or location in the colon. Distal colon is closer to the rectum. Proximal colon is closer to the cecum.

diverticula: Pouch-like sacks of the colon that can resemble polyps, but are not related to cancer.

diverticulitis: An inflammation of diverticula.

diverticulosis: Having a number of diverticula.

DNA: *Deoxyriboneucleic acid.* Material in the nucleus (brain of the cell) that codes what that cell will become, its job.

dysplasia: Abnormal growth of cells.

electrocautery: Surgical tool that utilizes electric current to cut and cauterize tissue. It is used to make incisions and to stem blood flow.

endoscopy: Visualization of a part of the gastrointestinal tract by a flexible instrument inserted into the gastrointestinal system.

enterocolitis: Another name for Crohn's disease.

Enterostomal therapist: Healthcare specialist trained to help patients care for and adjust to colostomy.

excisional biopsy: Surgical biopsy that removes entire lesion.

familial adenomatous polyposis (FAP): Inherited condition in which hundreds of polyps develop in the colon and rectum.

fecal occult blood test: Test to check for any blood that might be hidden in the stool.

flow cytometry: Analysis of tumor cells performed on biopsy specimens to determine the number of cells that are multiplying in order to try to determine how fast the tumor is growing.

flurouracil, 5-FU: Cytotoxic drug used to treat colon cancer.

FOBT: See fecal occult blood test.

Gardner's syndrome: A genetic colon condition similar to FAP.

gastroenterologist: An internist with additional training in digestive diseases, including training in endoscopy.

gene: Unit of heredity arranged on a chromosome. The polyposis gene is carried by chromosome 5.

general anesthesia: Drugs that cause complete unconsciousness during surgery.

genetic markers: Abnormalities found in the genes that indicate the potential for cancer.

hemicolectomy: Partial colectomy.

Hemoccult®: Type of occult fecal blood test.

hemorrhoid: Benign vascular growth commonly found in the anus.

histologic diagnosis: Study of what is under the microscope; the most minute branch of anatomic study; the information in your pathology report.

hyperplasia: Abnormal growth of cells.

ileostomy: Surgical formation of an opening in the abdominal wall through which the small intestine will be passed and feces will be emptied into a bag.

ileum: Small intestine.

infusion: The continuous, slow introduction of a drug through a vein.

in situ: A cancer that is "in place," noninvasive, and has not spread beyond that histologic structure.

intravenous: Medication entering the body by way of a vein.

invasive: Kind of cancer that can or has spread from its histologic original site.

irradiation: Radiation therapy.

irritable bowel syndrome: Condition similar to colitis, but not a risk factor for colon cancer.

J-pouch: A J-shaped new rectum made of the lower end of the small intestine, which is joined to the anus.

lesion: Tumor, mass, or other abnormality.

leucovorin: Chemotherapy medication used in combination with flurouracil (5-FU) in treating colon cancer.

levasimole: Chemotherapy medication used in combination with flurouracil (5-FU) in treating colon cancer.

local excision: Surgical procedure requiring only local anesthesia.

local treatment: Treatment aimed at the cells in the colon tumor and the area close to it.

local anesthesia: Drug that numbs only a particular area of the body.

lumen: Space inside the colon; the passageway.

lymph: Almost colorless fluid that travels through the lymphatic system, bathing body tissues and carrying cells that help fight infection; operates much like the circulatory system.

lymphatic system: Tissues and organs, including the bone marrow, spleen, thymus, and lymph nodes, that produce and store cells that fight infection and disease.

lymph nodes: Small, bean-shaped organs located along the lymphatic system. Nodes filter bacteria or cancer cells that might travel through the lymphatic system. Also called *lymph glands*.

lymphoma: Primary cancer of the lymph nodes.

magnetic resonance imaging (MRI): Radiologic study that utilizes a magnet to generate cross-sectional images of the body; gives excellent detail about soft tissue densities; used to detect bone cancer and other conditions, and to sometimes evaluate lymph nodes.

malignant: A cancerous condition.

margins of resection: Cut edges of the specimen taken out during biopsy; edges of the excision (excised tissue), such as a section of colon; checked for the presence of tumor cells. If no cancer has reached the edge of the tissue, margins are clean.

mass: Term used to describe a lesion, tumor, lump, nodule.

metachronous: Term used to describe a colonic polyp that occurs after the original polyp was found.

metastasis: Spread of cancer from one part of the body to another.

metastatic disease: Cancer that has spread from its original site to other parts of the body; most commonly bone, lung, liver, brain, lymph nodes.

206

metastatic lesions: Cancerous lesion or tumor at another site that has the same cancer cells as the original tumor.

microinvasive: Cancer that has less than 5 or 10 percent showing invasion. The rest is noninvasive.

micrometastasis: Less than 2 millimeters of metastasis in a lymph node.

m-rad: Unit of measure for radiation.

mucosa: Mucous membrane lining the inside of the colon; a membrane rich in mucous glands.

muscularis propria: Outer wall of the colon.

neoplasia: Proliferation of cells whose growth exceeds and is uncoordinated with other cells.

necrosis: Presence of dead cells.

negative nodes: Lymph nodes showing no signs of colon cancer.

noninvasive: In situ cancer that does not spread outside the polyp or colon lining.

occult cancer: Cancer that is hidden from view, not detectable by clinical methods alone.

oncogene: Gene that may promote cancer.

oncologist: Doctor who specializes in treating cancer; medical oncologist, surgical oncologist, radiation oncologist, etc.

palliative: Relieves symptoms such as pain; does not cure.

partial colectomy: See *colectomy*.

pathologic diagnosis: A histologic diagnosis, report on the state of the microscopic particles of the tumor.

pathologist: Doctor who identifies diseases by studying cells and tissues under a microscope.

pedunculated: Condition of adenoma having a stalk.

perfusion: Forcing a fluid through an organ, such as the liver, via the blood vessels.

permanent section: Final report after full pathologic evaluation; tissue removed during biopsy that is preserved for thorough study.

polyp: Small outgrowth of tissue arising from the mucous membrane of the colon.

polyposis: Disease involving the occurrence of multiple polyps in the colon and rectum.

port: Small device that is implanted under the skin with a catheter that enters the vessels of the chest and into which medications can be infused; infusaport.

positive lymph nodes: Lymph nodes that contain cancer cells.

premalignant: Condition that indicates a significant potential for cancer.

primary tumor: Original site of the colon cancer; the first.

proctocolectomy: Surgical removal of the colon and the entire rectum, including a permanent ileostomy.

proctosigmoidoscopy: Visualization of the rectum and lower sigmoid colon by an endoscope.

prognostic indicators: All elements of the disease used to determine prognosis and treatment, such as size and location of the tumor and behavior of the cells involved, number of nodes, patient's age, etc.

RTX: Medical shorthand for *radiation treatment*. Also XRT.

radiation oncologist: Physician who specializes in radiation treatment.

radiation therapy: Treatment with high-energy rays from X rays or other sources to kill or slow cancer cells; can also reduce pain from cancer spread to bone by killing tumor at this site.

rectum: Area at the end of the colon where fecal matter is stored until it is eliminated.

serosa: Thin membrane with cells that secrete fluid.

sigmoid colon: Portion of the colon located on the lower left side of the abdomen, between the descending colon and the rectum.

sigmoidoscopy: Examination of the rectum and lower colon using a sigmoidoscope.

sphincter muscles: Circular muscles at the exit point of the rectum and other parts of the digestive system that control the flow of matter through the system.

staging: Process of learning whether cancer has spread from its original site to another part of the body. Clinical stage is based upon history and physical examination. Pathologic stage is based upon finding under the microscope.

stoma: Surgically created opening into the body from the outside.

submucosa: Supporting layer of connective tissue directly under the mucosa, or the mucous membrane lining the colon.

synchronous: Appearing at the same time. *Metachronous* is at different times, maybe a year apart.

systemic therapy: Treatment that goes through the system, usually via the blood, and reaches and affects cells all over the body.

transverse colon: Portion of the colon that crosses the abdomen from right side to left side, near the navel.

tumor: Mass of tissue, lesion, lump, nodule.

Tx: Medical shorthand for *treatment*. Also *Rx*.

ultrasound: Diagnostic test that bounces sound waves off tissues and converts the echoes into pictures.

INDEX

211

ABOUT THE AUTHORS

Paul Miskovitz is a gastroenterologist who guides patients through the diagnosis of colon cancer, helps them understand treatment options, and supervises follow-up care. He has written many professional papers and a medical book chapter on colon cancer.

Dr. Miskovitz did his internship and residency at The New York Hospital-Cornell Medical Center and has been a member of the Division of Digestive Diseases there since 1978. He is a clinical associate professor of medicine at Cornell Medical College and associate attending physician at The New York Hospital. Dr. Miskovitz serves on many professional boards and committees and is known for his teaching activity at Cornell Medical College.

He has been on the hospital's Food and Nutrition advisory committee since 1988 and is a member of the hospital's quality assurance committee. His research activities have included participation in the Memorial Sloan-Kettering Cancer Center Colonic Polyp Prevention Trial. Dr. Miskovitz maintains an office in Manhattan.

Marian Betancourt has been a professional writer and editor for more than 20 years. Her work has appeared in national magazines and newspapers. Since 1990, she has written extensively about medical issues. She is coauthor of *What to Do if You Get Breast Cancer,* published in 1995, and *Chronic Illness and the Family: A Guide for Living Every Day,* published in March 1996. A book about prostate cancer will be published in 1998. She is also writing a book about domestic violence for HarperCollins. Betancourt is a member of the American Society of Journalists and Authors, the Author's Guild, and the Authors Registry. She lives in Brooklyn, New York.